HEALTH CARE CAREERS IN 2 YEARS™

JUMP-STARTING A CAREER IN DENTISTRY

CAROL HAND

I0808589

Rosen YA™
New York

Published in 2019 by The Rosen Publishing Group, Inc.
29 East 21st Street, New York, NY 10010

First Edition

Library of Congress Cataloging-in-Publication Data

Names: Hand, Carol, 1945– author.
Title: Jump-starting a career in dentistry / Carol Hand.
Description: New York: Rosen Young Adult, 2019. | Series: Health care careers in 2 years | Audience: Grades 7–12. | Includes bibliographical references and index.
Identifiers: LCCN 2018002636| ISBN 9781508184966 (library bound) | ISBN 9781508184959 (pbk.)
Subjects: LCSH: Dentistry—Vocational guidance—Juvenile literature. | Dentist—Juvenile literature.
Classification: LCC RK60 .H36 2019 | DDC 617.6/0233—dc23
LC record available at https://lccn.loc.gov/2018002636

Manufactured in the United States of America

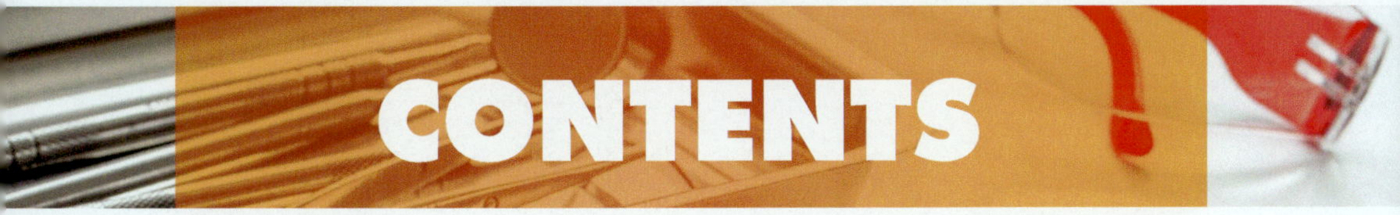

CONTENTS

INTRODUCTION

Karen Siebert is a dental hygienist. According to her description of a day in her life on the job, posted online at the College of Lake County in Illinois, her day starts early and involves more than just cleaning teeth. She begins about half an hour before her first patient arrives. She reviews the charts of that day's patients, looking at what treatment they need, their past health history, and the date and reason for their last visit. In her treatment room, Siebert checks to see that all surfaces are clean and the room is stocked with supplies. She sets out the instruments needed for her first patient. Today, she will see six patients. The length of each appointment varies according to what the patient needs done. Two adults and two children are coming for preventive appointments. These will be about an hour each. Two others are being treated for gum disease. Their appointments will last for about ninety minutes.

Because patients are often fearful or uncomfortable in a dentist's office, Siebert is friendly and welcoming. She asks about her patients' lives, families, and jobs. Education is also an important part of dental hygiene. Siebert always spends a few minutes with each patient discussing how they can take better care of their teeth at home. She reviews and updates the patient's health history. If necessary, she takes a digital X-ray, which the

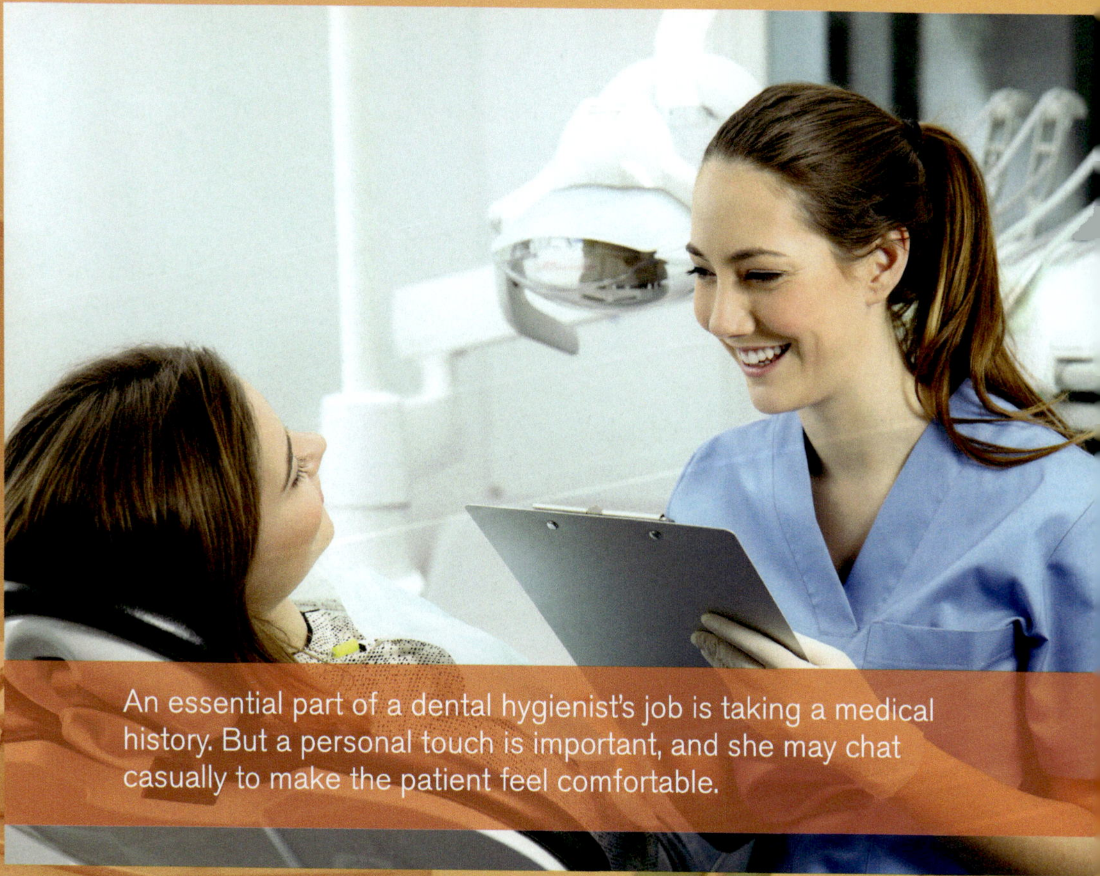

An essential part of a dental hygienist's job is taking a medical history. But a personal touch is important, and she may chat casually to make the patient feel comfortable.

patient can view on the computer screen. Before proceeding to the treatment portion of the appointment, she dons disposable gloves, mask, and eye protection. She begins with an examination of the patient's teeth and gums, carefully noting all her observations in the computer and on the patient's chart. This note taking ensures that the dentist, who will visit for only about five minutes during the appointment, has all the information needed for the patient's treatment. Then, Siebert scales the patient's teeth to remove plaque and polishes them. When finished, she makes sure the patient understands what future treatment is necessary and schedules an appointment.

After the patient leaves, Siebert returns to clean and disinfect the room. This essential step prevents passing infections from one patient to another. She follows a similar sequence for all patients. For patients with gum disease, she uses special instruments to help remove infectious bacteria. She may even administer a local anesthetic if she must remove diseased tissue. She spends seven to eight hours per day with patients, with an hour break for lunch. When the last patient leaves, Siebert must clean and disinfect the treatment room, including the floor. She inspects all instruments and prepares them for sterilizing. She places them in the sterilizer and turns it on before she leaves. The next day, she starts over with a new group of patients.

Dental hygienist is one of several dentistry jobs, including dental assistant and dental laboratory technician, that can be learned in two to three years or fewer. Siebert finds it fun and rewarding. She feels a sense of pride in helping people maintain good dental health for a lifetime. She especially likes getting to know her patients. "The more you know them, the more you can help them," she says.

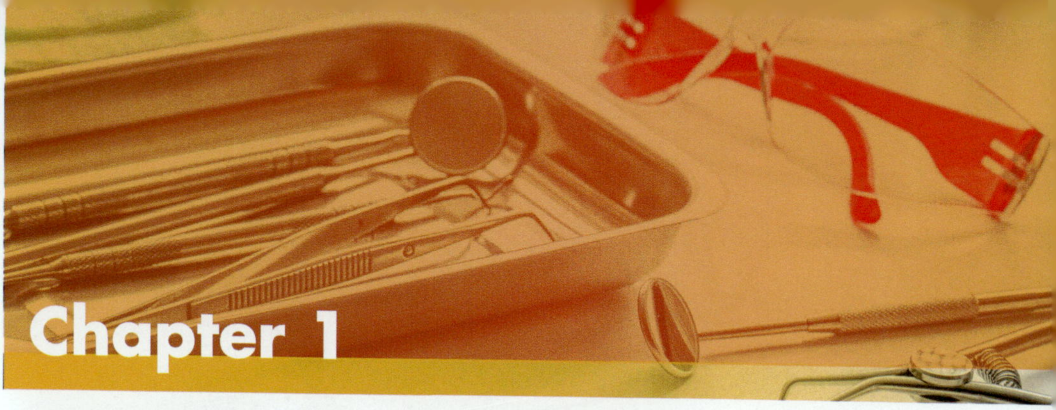

Chapter 1

BEING A DENTAL ASSISTANT

Dental assistants play a key role in any dental office. Their tasks and responsibilities vary by office and by state. But primarily, their job is to assist the dentist in whatever ways are needed, from caring for patients to caring for dental instruments to scheduling appointments. They ensure that the dental office runs smoothly. They work closely with patients, making sure they are comfortable, informed, and well cared for. Most dental assistants consider this one-on-one interaction with patients the best part of their job.

A Day in the Life

A dental assistant's day starts early. Dental assistants usually arrive at least a half-hour before the first patient's appointment and set up the office for the day. This procedure involves making sure all dental chairs are stocked with equipment and supplies and charts for all the day's patients are pulled and ready for the dentist or dental hygienist to view. Administrative or clerical duties are often an important part of the dental assistant's day.

Assistants may schedule appointments, code insurance bills, or process patient invoices and payments. They may work directly with patients to handle any problems with scheduling or payments.

Before the appointment, dental assistants seat the patient in the chair and make sure they are comfortable. They discuss upcoming procedures, answer any questions, and reassure the patient. They may be asked to update the patient's medical history and record new information on the chart or in the computer. During exams or procedures, the dental assistant may work with the hygienist and dentist, handing them the proper tools. They may use the suction hose to keep the patient's mouth clean and dry or rinse the patient's mouth during and after a procedure.

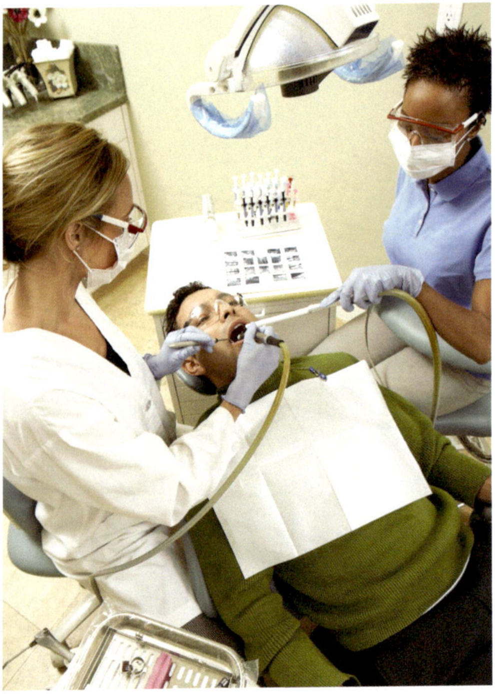

A dental assistant helps the dentist or hygienist in whatever is needed, including suctioning. Both professionals must wear protective gear, including gloves and face masks.

After the appointment, the dental assistant may answer the patient's questions about care of the person's teeth at home and give practical tips on good dental hygiene. One of the assistant's most important jobs is to ensure that the patient has a

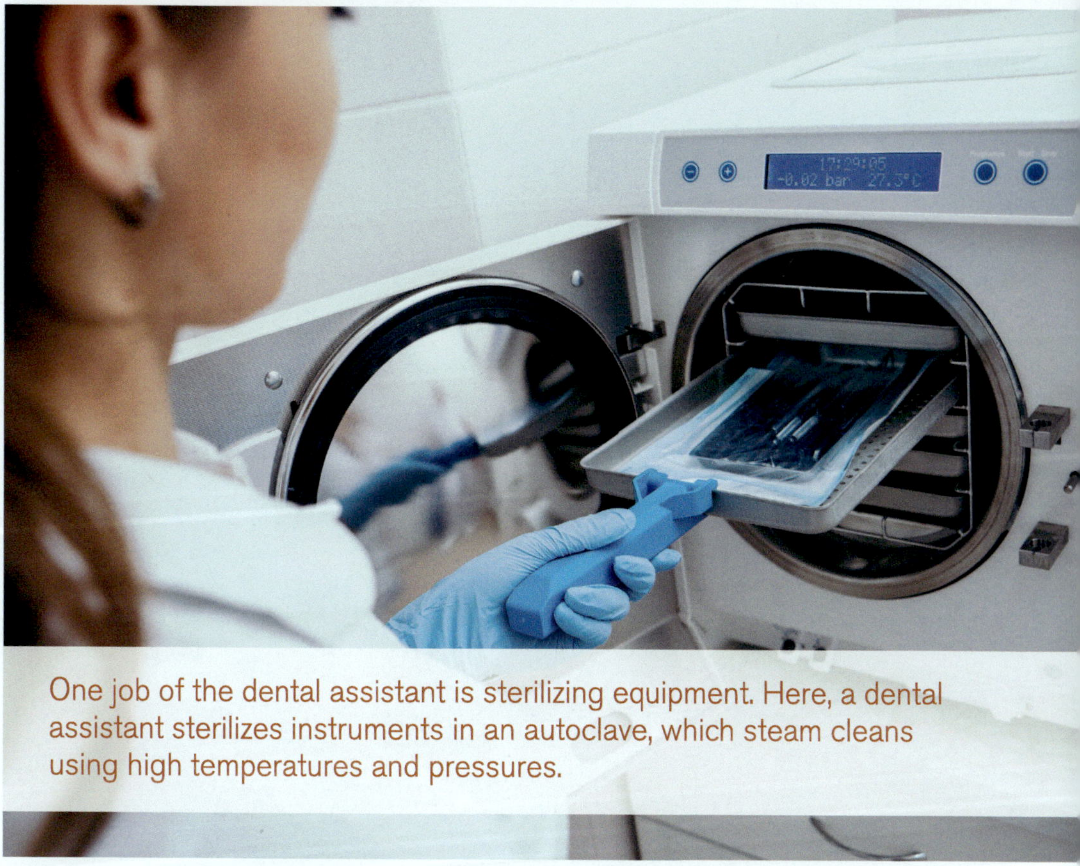

One job of the dental assistant is sterilizing equipment. Here, a dental assistant sterilizes instruments in an autoclave, which steam cleans using high temperatures and pressures.

positive experience and leaves the office feeling good about the appointment.

In addition to direct interactions with patients and other dental staff members, dental assistants may have additional routine responsibilities throughout the day. They call patients to confirm appointments and send out reminder cards. They order and restock supplies and clean and disinfect dental offices between patients. They make sure the dentist has the appropriate equipment needed for upcoming patients. They sterilize equipment. Depending on the office (or the state in which they practice), they may also take and process X-rays and perform laboratory

DENTAL ASSISTANTS—ALWAYS ON THE MOVE

Michelle Schooley became a dental assistant because she had always had dental problems and wanted to help other people with similar problems. Schooley discovered that dental assisting keeps her extremely busy, but it's never monotonous. She may see dozens of patients each day. Dental assistants rarely sit down, she says. They are constantly in motion. When she arrives, Schooley prepares the office for the day. For each patient and procedure, she must prepare about twenty different things. These duties include bringing the patient to the dentist's chair, seating the patient, and putting on a bib. In a busy office, multiple patients are being seen simultaneously. This activity usually means she is running from room to room. She might seat and prepare a patient in one room, help the dentist or hygienist in another, and clean and restock a third room after the patient has left. Jaime Owen, writing about Schooley's career on Aol.com, quotes Michelle as saying, "There's always a different tooth, a different patient. You have the same procedures, but it's always a different task."

tests. They may polish teeth, apply sealants or fluoride, apply topical anesthetics to a patient's mouth before a procedure, or remove sutures after a procedure.

Personal Qualities

A good dental assistant must have a variety of personal qualities. These include dexterity and attention to detail. Dental assistants work with their hands. They must be able to use tools precisely, as they work in close quarters and in a small area of the patient's body—the mouth. They must use their detail skills to carry out precise rules and protocols, such as infection control and sterilization procedures. They must be aware of which procedures they are

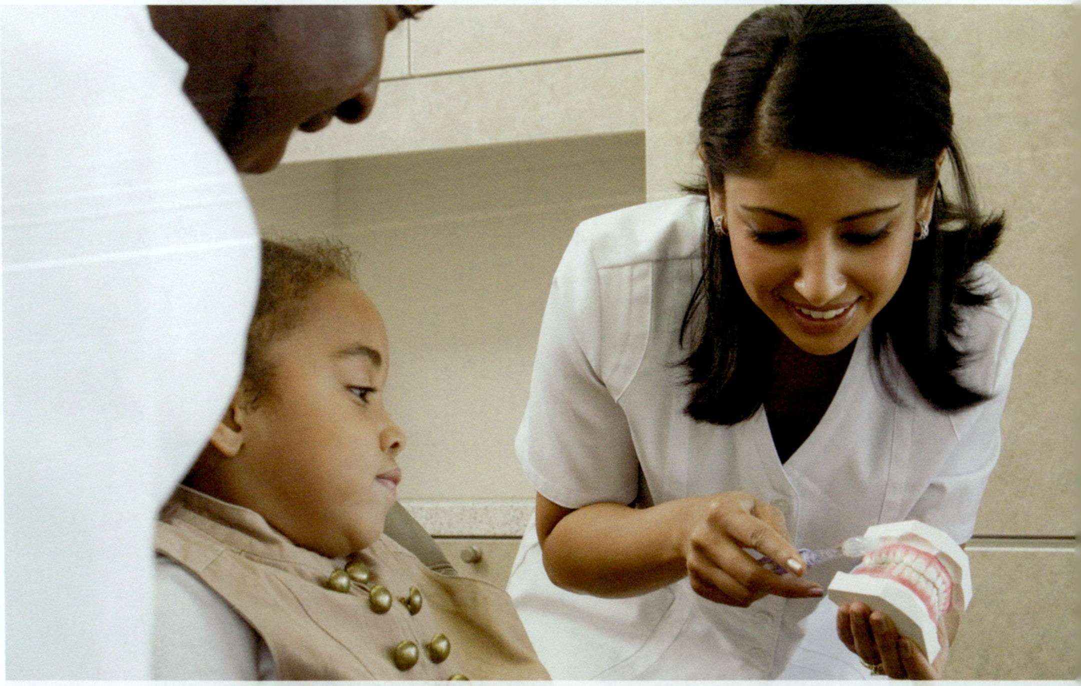

Practicing good dental care prevents cavities and ensures more pleasant dental visits. Here, a dental assistant uses a model to teach a young patient proper brushing techniques.

and are not allowed to perform. Good dental assistants also need good organizational skills. This ability will help them prepare patient trays with the correct instruments and supplies. It will also be useful in maintaining patient records, organizing appointments and payments, and ordering supplies.

Perhaps the most important skills a dental assistant must have are people skills. Dental assistants work very closely with patients and therefore must be sensitive to their emotional needs. Many patients fear dental procedures, so they need reassurance. Dental assistants can provide a calming influence and can impart information about the procedure, so the patient knows what to expect. They should be mindful of whether the patient is in pain and make the dentist and hygienist aware of this discomfort, so they can address the pain. In addition, dental assistants must be good listeners. They must listen not only to patients, but to others in the practice. Dentists and hygienists give them instructions for carrying out procedures (for example, taking X-rays or sterilizing equipment), which they must follow to the letter.

Techniques and Technology

Dental assistants participate in a variety of procedures, including exams, cleanings, fillings, root canals, and dental surgery. They are required to use specialized equipment to assist with these procedures. The air-water syringe is a metal device that attaches to both an air and a water supply. It consists of a long, thin tube and two buttons, one for air and one for water. Dental assistants use the air button to blow away debris and saliva that obscure the dentist's field of view. They use the water button for rinsing when the dentist fills a cavity or seals a tooth.

The saliva ejector (also called a spit-suction device) is used during most procedures. It has a handle attached to a flexible tube, which in turn is attached to the suction device. It allows the dental assistant to remove excess saliva from the mouth. This removal is essential, because the patient often cannot swallow during a procedure. The high-volume evacuator is similar to the saliva ejector, with a wider-diameter tube. It is often used during dental surgery, root canals, or fillings to remove large pieces of tooth or food. If not removed,

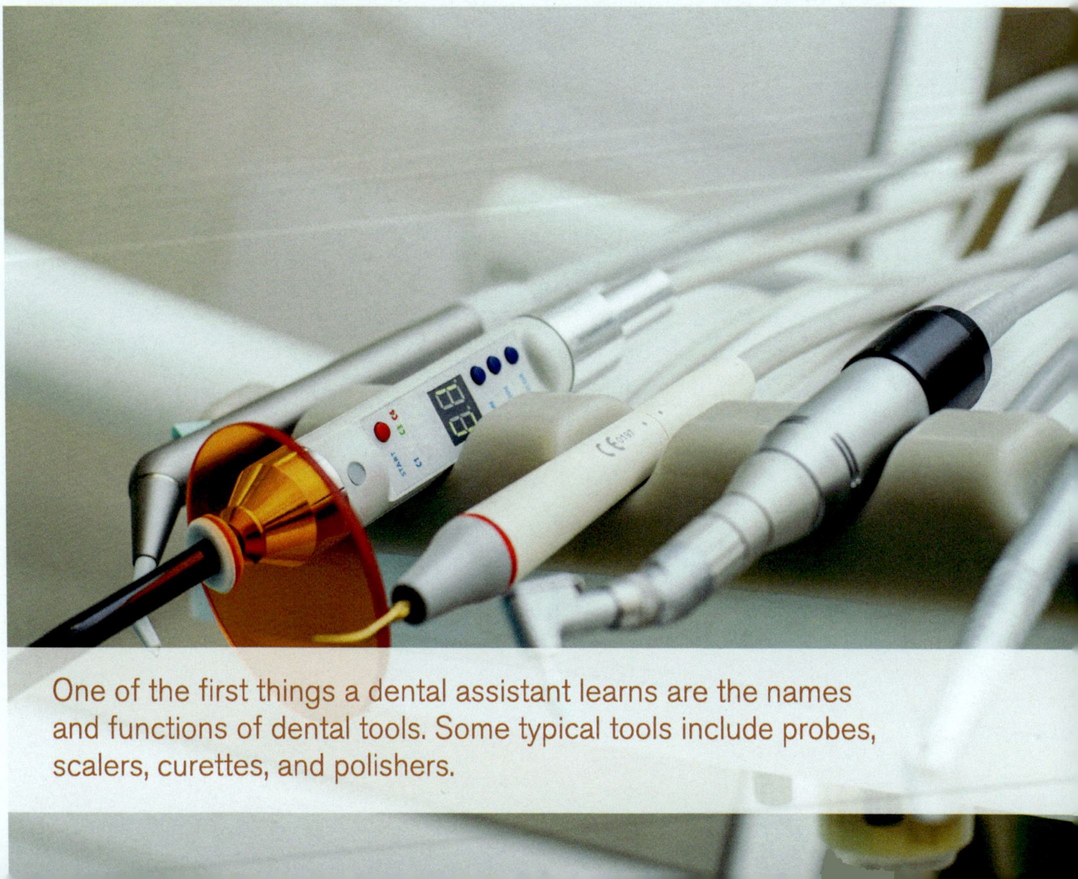

One of the first things a dental assistant learns are the names and functions of dental tools. Some typical tools include probes, scalers, curettes, and polishers.

these could result in infections or prevent the procedure from being completed properly.

In addition, dental assistants must know the names and functions of the various tools used in the dental office. They will be required to hand these tools to the dentist or hygienist during procedures. They will also need to sterilize them, using specialized procedures, every day. In some dental offices, dental assistants will need to become familiar with the correct use and care of the X-ray machine. Much of this information will be learned or perfected during on-the-job training. For workplace safety, a dental assistant who operates an X-ray machine should wear a personal dosimeter badge (a device that monitors radiation levels in an area) to ensure that he or she has not been exposed to radiation.

Training and Benefits

Dental assisting is the easiest and fastest dental field to enter. In some states, only a high school diploma is required. These assistants learn by on-the-job training. They are taught by another dental assistant, a dental hygienist, or a dentist in the office where they work. But most dental assistants take a special course from an accredited program.

Community colleges, vocational or technical schools, or colleges and university dental schools offer accredited programs in dental assisting. Some programs are accelerated, part time, or long distance. Programs usually last one year or less and result in a diploma or certificate. Accredited programs are recognized and approved by the Commission on Dental Accreditation (CODA), part of the American Dental Association (ADA). CODA accredits approximately 270 programs in the United States. In the one-year program, students do classroom and laboratory training. They learn about the mouth, jaws, teeth, and gums and about the tools used in dentistry. Near the end of the course, they do a practical course, or practicum, in which they practice the skills they have learned under supervision. Two-year programs are less common. They result in an associate's degree, such as an associate of applied science (AAS), which includes general education, technical training, and longer clinical practicums.

Most states do not require a dental assistant to be certified at the entry level, but they require a license or certification to advance. Usually, specific licenses are required to work in specialties such as radiography (X-ray) or infection control. Certification, which requires passing a test, is conducted by the Dental Assisting National Board (DANB).

The Bureau of Labor Statistics (BLS), an agency within the US Department of Labor, regularly updates the *Occupational Outlook Handbook*, a reference that supplies career information, including training and education, pay, and job prospects for the future, for countless occupations. In October 2017, the BLS reported a median salary of $37,000 per year for dental assistants. The job outlook is excellent. Employment is expected to grow 19 percent between 2016 and 2026, according to the BLS. As dental care continues to improve and people keep more of their teeth longer, the need for preventive care will increase.

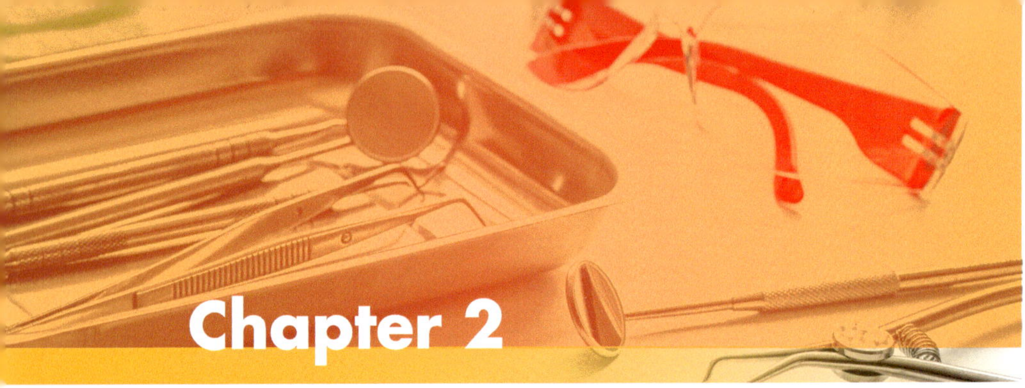

Chapter 2

BEING A DENTAL LABORATORY TECHNICIAN

Sometimes a dental patient needs more than just a cleaning or filling. Sometimes one or more teeth must be pulled and replaced with a crown, bridge, or even dentures. Perhaps a young patient needs braces. When dental work requires new structures to be inserted into the mouth, it's time to call for the help of dental laboratory technicians. These dental professionals are responsible for measuring, modeling, and constructing new dental appliances.

What Dental Lab Technicians Do

Dental lab technicians (DLTs), also called dental lab assistants, seldom work directly with patients. They work in laboratories associated with dental offices. They work closely with dentists or orthodontists (dentists who use braces to correct irregular teeth). Some DLTs work alone in a lab with a single dentist. Others contract out, working for various dentists as needed. Still others work in large labs, as members of a group of DLTs. Those who work in small offices may do all laboratory activities, while those in larger labs often specialize.

When a patient needs a new dental appliance, the dentist or orthodontist makes a mold of the patient's teeth. Sometimes, instead of a physical mold, the prescription or work order includes a digital rendering of the patient's teeth. The dental lab technician uses the mold to make a wax replica of the teeth and then uses the replica to build the new appliance. The technician bends, grinds, and shapes the material. This process involves building layers of porcelain or other material, polishing and smoothing the appliance, and checking the bite. The dentist takes the new appliance for a fitting and may bring it back several times until it is comfortable and precisely fits the patient's mouth. An exact fit is essential, or the appliance will not work well or look natural. Dental lab technicians may help dentists decide on the best type of material to use for the appliance. They may also repair existing dental

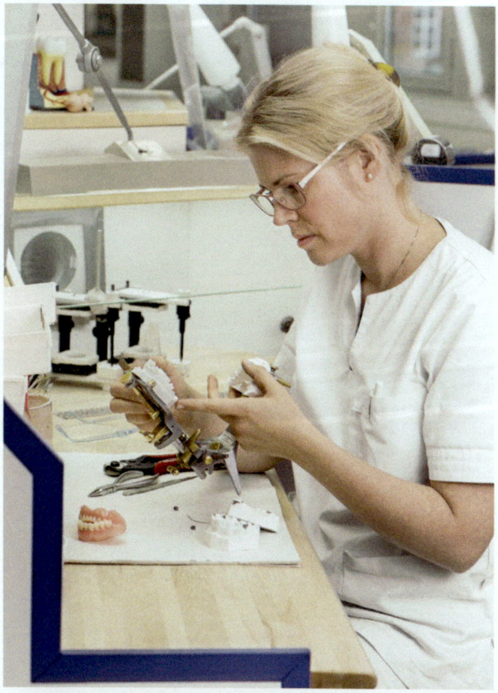

Dental lab technicians design dentures by working with wax molds or digital representations of a patient's mouth. Here, a dental technician assembles a set of dentures.

appliances. For example, they might rebuild denture linings or repair retainers (the part of an appliance, such as a bridge or brace, used to hold it in place).

Dental laboratory technicians may develop one or more specialties. Two general groups of specialties include restorative dentistry (prosthodontics) and orthodontics. Prosthodontics involves the creation of appliances including full dentures to replace all of a person's teeth, removable partial dentures or fixed bridges to replace several missing teeth, crowns (caps to cover teeth and restore them to their original size and shape), veneers to improve appearance and function, or implants. Orthodontics involves the creation of night guards, braces, and splints to straighten, align, and protect teeth. Movement of a person's teeth through orthodontics improves both the function and appearance of the teeth and mouth. Each restoration a dental lab technician makes is unique to the patient. A good technician recreates both the perfection and the imperfections of the person's teeth to provide an appliance that is not only functional, but looks natural.

Personal Qualities, Techniques, and Technologies

The work of a dental lab technician is solitary; the person must be able to work well alone. The work is also delicate and painstaking, requiring attention to detail, excellent hand-eye coordination, and color perception. DLTs must be able to use small tools and instruments and manipulate many kinds of dental materials. They must be able to make minor

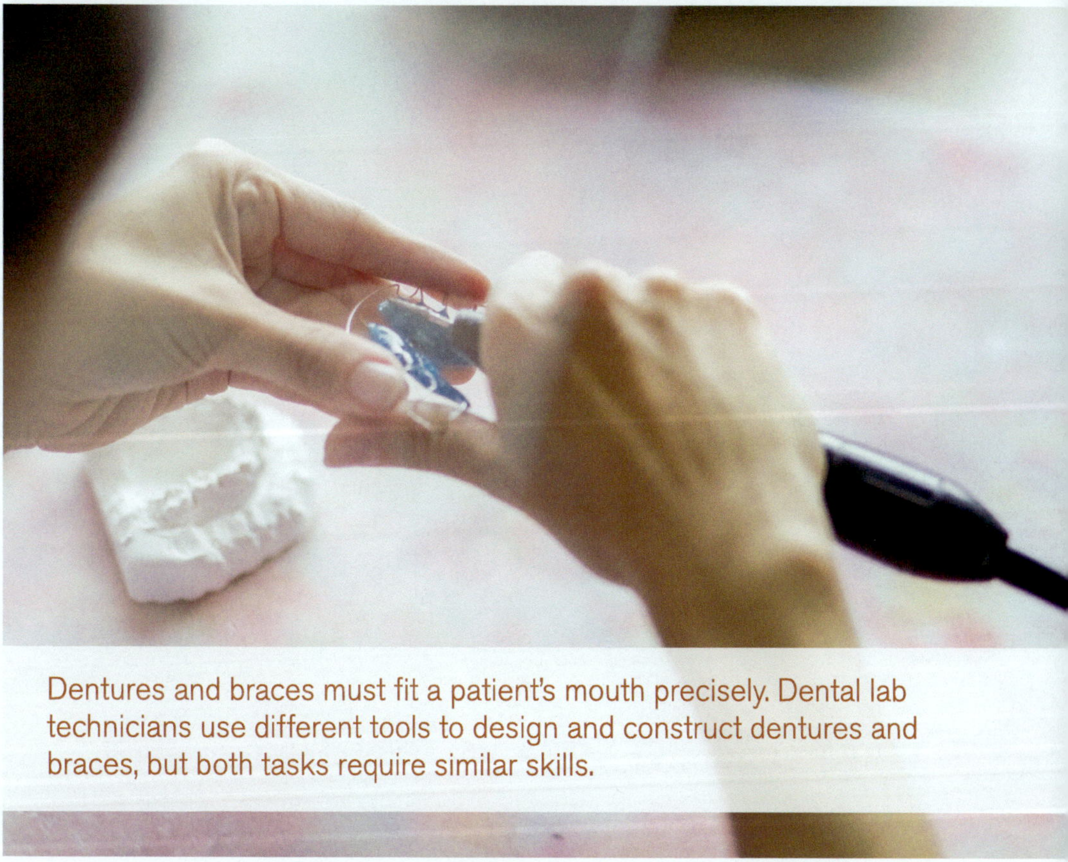

Dentures and braces must fit a patient's mouth precisely. Dental lab technicians use different tools to design and construct dentures and braces, but both tasks require similar skills.

adjustments quickly, to produce an exact fit for the patient. A dental lab technician's work combines art and science. Although he or she must understand both dental science and materials science, the work also requires many of the skills of a sculptor and an eye for drawing and design.

Dental prosthetics (artificial structures) are made from a variety of different materials. Dental lab technicians must work with waxes, metal alloys, stainless steel, and different kinds of porcelains, plastics, and glass polymers. They must understand the distinctions among these materials and be

NEW TRENDS IN BRACES

At one time, teens and preteens dreaded getting braces. Braces were uncomfortable, even painful, and they carried a social stigma. But times have changed. Gone are most heavy metal brackets. New materials and methods can produce straight, beautiful teeth with much less pain, often in a shorter amount of time. Even adults who missed out on tooth straightening in childhood are joining the trend.

Clear braces are similar to the original metal brackets and wires but are much less visible. The brackets are tooth-colored rather than clear, and they allow treatment of even severe misalignments. Clear aligners are truly clear. They slide over the person's own teeth and are nearly undetectable. They are excellent for treating minor orthodontic problems. With 3D digital images, dentists can show patients the progress of their orthodontic experience. Patients can see what the final outcome will look like. This perspective can serve as a powerful motivator for completing the process.

Several trends are combining to decrease the length of the orthodontic process. Braces can be made right in the dentist's office,

using new compact and efficient machines. The National Aeronautics and Space Administration (NASA) has developed a heat-activated metal that changes shape with mouth temperature. Braces made with this metal change shape slowly between adjustments, so teeth align faster and braces can be removed more quickly. For people most concerned with cosmetic changes, a new process can straighten teeth so they are nearly perfect in six months, instead of the usual two years. Finally, kids can now flaunt their braces, rather than hiding them. They can turn orthodontic appliances into fashion accessories by choosing, for example, fluorescent, glow-in-the-dark braces.

able to determine which will work best for each appliance. They manipulate these materials using a variety of small hand tools, including files, wax carvers and spatulas, small knives, small hand drills, and polishers. They also use computer programs and 3D printers to receive impressions from the consulting dentist and to create the actual appliances.

Training and Benefits

Many dental laboratory technicians learn by on-the-job training. They begin with very simple tasks, such as pouring material into impressions, and work up to more complicated tasks, such as making dentures or bridges or bending wires for braces. Complete on-the-job training takes three to four years, but it may take several more years for a technician to be considered an expert. Dental lab technicians can also receive formal training through community colleges, vocational or technical institutes, or the military. Most programs take two years, and include courses in dental anatomy, denture-making techniques, and dental casting (converting a wax impression into a finished dental appliance). These courses include considerable lab work. Programs may also include courses in industrial safety and professional ethics. Degree programs (such as associate's degrees) will also include general studies classes. Certification for dental technicians is available through the National Board for Certification in Dental Laboratory Technology (NBC). Applicants must pass three tests: a comprehensive test and a practical and a written exam for at least one specialty. There are five possible specialties: complete dentures, removable partial dentures, crown and bridge, ceramics, and orthodontics. Technicians may choose to pursue certification

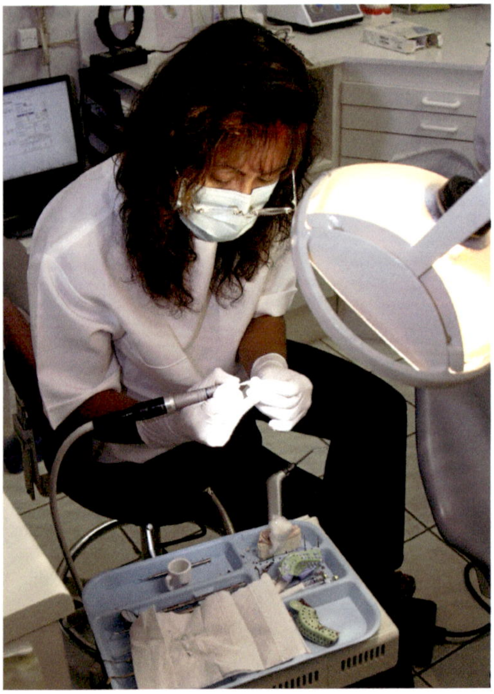

Because they handle materials that go in a patient's mouth, dental lab technicians must work in a very clean laboratory environment. They must also wear protective gear.

in several specialties. Some dentists will hire technicians only if they are certified.

The BLS reported in October 2017 that the mean salary for a certified dental laboratory technician was $37,680. Jobs in this field are projected to grow by 13 percent between 2016 and 2026; thus, the job outlook is good. Most dental laboratory technicians work in commercial dental laboratories that typically employ between five and ten people (although a few are much larger, employing up to two hundred). Some laboratories produce a full range of dental prosthetics; others specialize in one, such as dentures or braces. Other technicians work in private dentists' offices, hospitals, or dental schools. There are also some opportunities in the military.

Because of the delicate duties involved, dental laboratory technicians work in clean, well-lighted, well-ventilated laboratories. They typically have their own workbench and tools, which sometimes include computer design software, scanners, and milling or printing equipment. Most work full-time (at least forty hours per week, often more if the technician is self-employed). More experienced dental lab assistants may choose either to move from a smaller to a larger lab or to strike out on their own. They may buy an existing shop, start their own, or become a private contractor, working with specific dentists or health maintenance organizations (HMOs). Dental laboratory technician is the only dental assistance field that gives its practitioners the option of starting their own business.

The dental laboratory technician field is wide open and primed to grow in the coming years. For a person with the right skills, it is an excellent career choice.

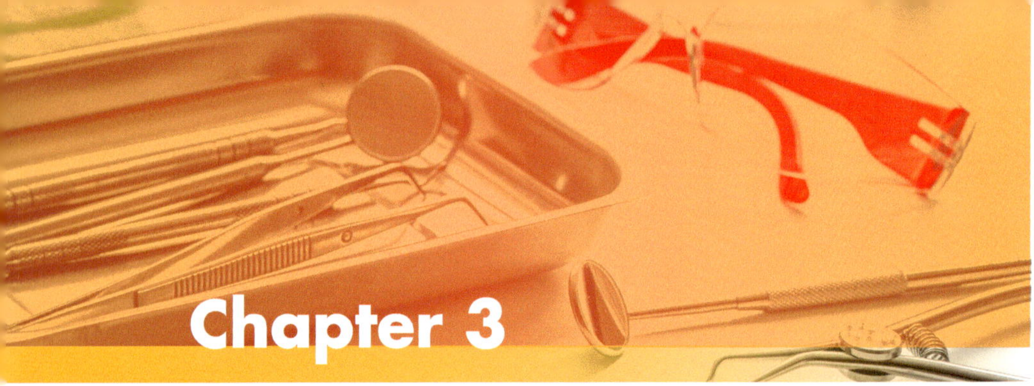

Chapter 3

BEING A DENTAL HYGIENIST

Kelli Swanson Jaecks, president of the American Dental Hygienists' Association in 2014 to 2015, likens dental hygienists to insurance agents. In the *U.S. News & World Report*'s review of best jobs, Jaecks points out that people see dentists when they have problems with their teeth, but they see dental hygienists to prevent those problems. A dentist may fill a cavity, do a root canal, or make a mold for a bridge or denture. Patients may fear visits to the dentist or at least not enjoy them. In contrast, a visit to a dental hygienist can be a very positive experience, because the patient is protecting his or her teeth. The hygienist cleans and treats the patient's teeth to keep them as healthy as possible—thereby decreasing the need for invasive procedures used by dentists to fix diseased or damaged teeth.

What Dental Hygienists Do

While dental hygienists work closely with dentists to keep patients' teeth healthy, they also work one on one with patients. For any given patient, their responsibilities might include screening procedures (such as review of the patient's health history, visual inspection of the teeth and mouth, completion of a dental chart, and taking blood pressure and pulse); taking and developing dental X-rays; cleaning the teeth (removing both hard and soft deposits, or tartar and plaque); applying sealants or fluorides to the teeth; and educating the patient on proper oral hygiene and the relation of good nutrition to dental health. Depending on the needs of the dental office, the hygienist may have other duties, from stocking supplies to administering local anesthetics.

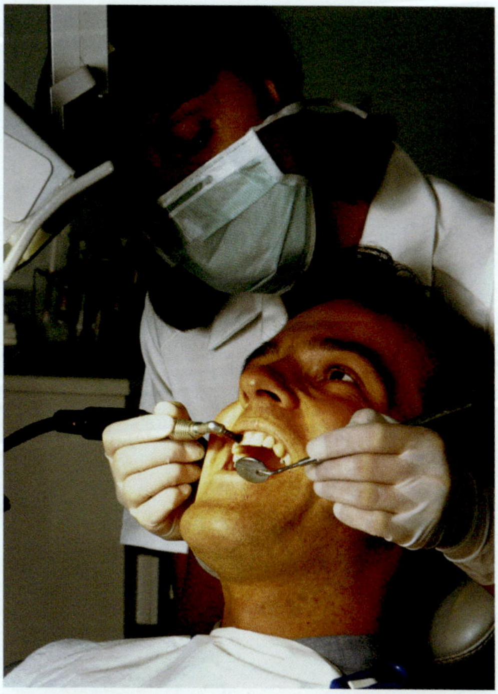

Polishing a patient's teeth removes stains and plaque, smooths the tooth surfaces, and makes teeth look more attractive. It is a vital part of a dental hygienist's job.

As professionals, dental hygienists must meet certain standards of dress and appearance to maintain the safety and health of both patient and hygienist. Because the hygienist works face to face with patients, it is important to prevent infections caused by exchange of germs. The dental hygienist always wears personal protective equipment (PPE). This PPE consists of a full-body plastic "barrier jacket," a plastic bonnet to cover the head, a face mask and a face shield or eye protection, and booties. Finally, the hygienist washes his or her hands and puts on surgical gloves. Typically, female hygienists also keep their hair pinned up away from their faces; they wear no jewelry and keep their nails short, with no artificial nails or polish.

Dental hygienists usually mention two things when describing why they love their jobs. First is the interaction with patients. They try to develop a friendly and trusting relationship with every patient, using their excellent communication skills to make patients feel comfortable and at ease, and to educate patients on maintaining their dental health. Thus, the field attracts those who love working with people. Second is the variety and flexibility of the job. Many love the fact that every patient is different, allowing them to develop relationships with many kinds of people. Some choose to specialize in working with certain groups of people, for example, children or the elderly. Many dental hygienists work full time, forty or more hours per week, but part-time positions are also available, some with evening and weekend hours. Although some hygienists work for individual dental practices, others work for community or educational institutions, dental corporations, or even in research. A potential downside is that, although not very stressful, the hygienist's job does require physical stamina. Hygienists are on their feet all day, often bending over, and may eventually develop back problems. Dental hygienists are at some risk of getting carpal tunnel syndrome because of the repetitious use of small dental tools.

In addition to an outgoing, friendly personality, dental hygienists must be detail oriented and have excellent manual dexterity and hand-eye coordination. These skills are

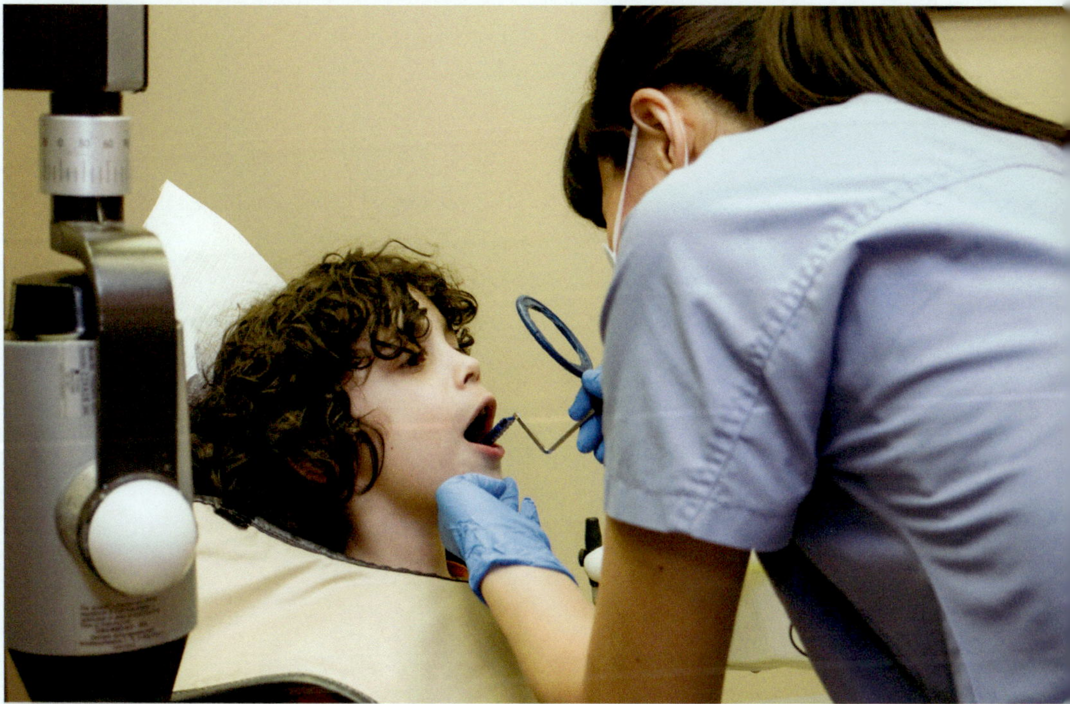

A dental hygienist prepares a patient for X-rays. The patient is covered with a lead apron, which will protect him from radiation as the X-rays are done.

especially important as they work with small (sometimes sharp) tools in the enclosed and delicate mouths of their patients. Critical-thinking skills will be valuable as they examine patients and make judgments regarding their dental health. For example, do patients appear to be brushing and flossing regularly? Do they show signs of incipient gum disease or cavities? Do they show signs of cancer or other abnormalities? The scope of the duties dental hygienists can carry out varies somewhat from state to state. But they are vital and respected members of the dental health team.

Tools and Technologies

Dental hygienists work with tool kits that include nearly twenty different hand instruments. These fall into several categories. Small, circular, handheld mirrors are important for seeing hard-to-reach spaces within the mouth, when the hygienist is checking for cavities or tartar. A probe is a metal instrument with a hooked shape and a sharp point. Probes are used for checking gum health and measuring depth of the pockets between teeth and gums. Each type of probe is specialized for a slightly different function. Scalers are pointed metal instruments used to scrape plaque and tartar off the tooth surfaces.

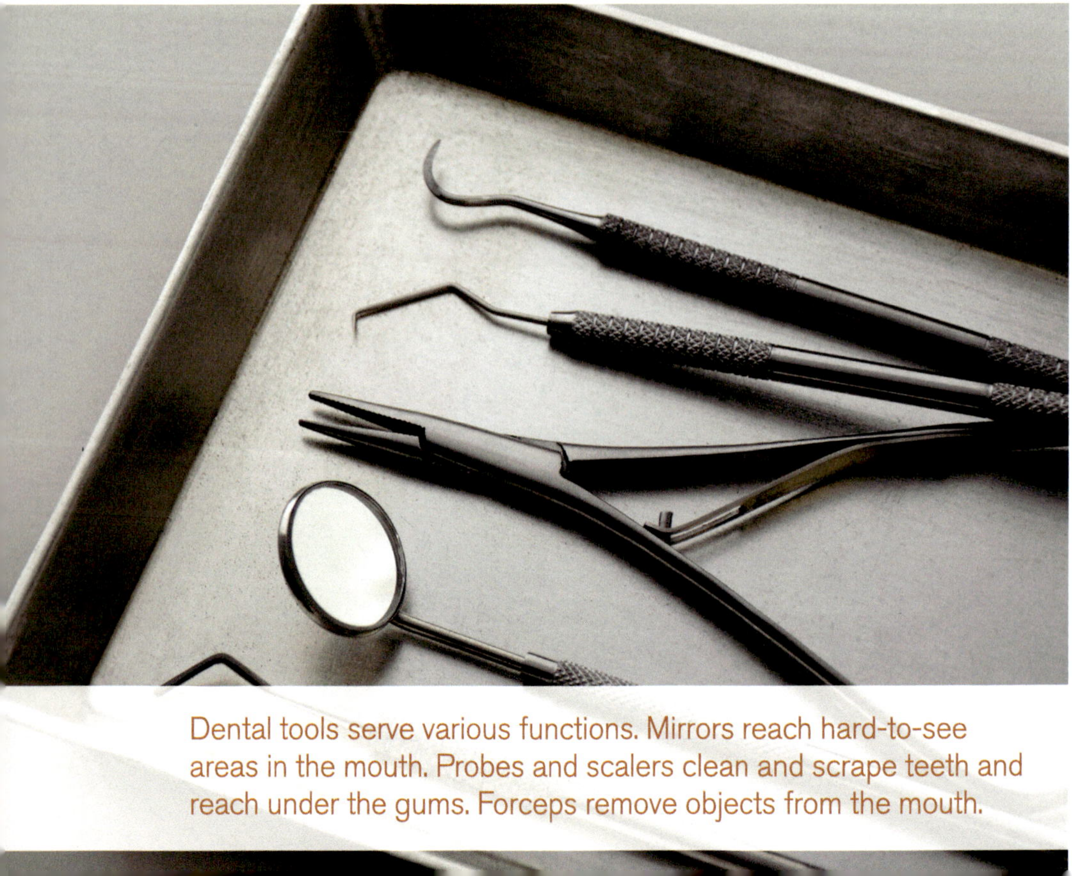

Dental tools serve various functions. Mirrors reach hard-to-see areas in the mouth. Probes and scalers clean and scrape teeth and reach under the gums. Forceps remove objects from the mouth.

Curettes are pointed metal instruments with rounded tips. They are used to scrape tartar from beneath the gums. Polishers are brushes used as finishing tools, used after the plaque and tartar are removed. Polishers spray on a polish that removes surface stains, buffs the teeth, and makes them shinier, much as a shoeshine brightens a pair of shoes. Their high rotation speed makes them very effective. Most dental hygienists now use ultrasonic scalers to remove tartar and stains.

ULTRASONICS IN DENTAL HYGIENE

At first, dental hygienists did all cleanings using only hand tools. But in the modern dental office, they often use ultrasonic scalers. Ultrasonic, or "beyond sound," refers to wavelengths of more than 15,000 hertz (Hz), or vibrations per second—above human hearing. Ultrasonic scalers consist of a medical device that emits an electrical signal and is attached to a handpiece by a cord. Various tool tips (scalers, files, polishers, and so on) can be fixed interchangeably to the end of the handheld device. The handpiece contains a piezoelectric transducer, composed of ceramic or quartz crystals, which transforms the electrical signal into ultrasonic vibrations.

(continued on the next page)

(continued from the previous page)

(Piezoelectric refers to electricity generated by pressure.) The vibrations are transmitted to the tool tip, which cleans the teeth. A piezoelectric scaler generates vibrations up to 50,000 Hz. A second type of ultrasonic scaler uses changing magnetic fields to generate the vibrations. These devices generate vibrations up to 25,000 Hz. Ultrasonic scalers clean teeth using cavitation, or the formation of tiny bubbles filled with water vapor rather than air. The vibrations stretch and compress the bubbles, causing them to implode. This implosion releases a tiny burst of heat and pressure that loosens particles stuck on the teeth. Water simultaneously cools the teeth, resulting in a painless and nonstressful procedure.

Ultrasonic scalers have no cutting edge, and patients usually find them comfortable to use. They have exchangeable tips that can remove deposits both above and below the gumline.

In addition, hygienists often remove some plaque with simple dental floss. They keep the mouth clean using a saliva ejector to suction out contaminants and excess saliva. They may use the air-water syringe to dry the teeth when necessary or to rinse out polish or contaminants. Dental hygienists must also be able to use the X-ray machine. Although not necessary for all patients, X-rays are essential for detecting decay or abnormalities in hidden areas. They provide information beyond that possible by visual inspection alone.

Training, Benefits, and Work Environment

Unlike dental assistants, who can begin their careers through on-the-job training, dental hygienists must have an associate's degree, which usually takes three years. Dental hygienist programs must be accredited by the Commission on Dental Accreditation of the American Dental Association. In 2015, the CODA accredited more than three hundred programs. Associate-level degrees are the most common, but some hygienists

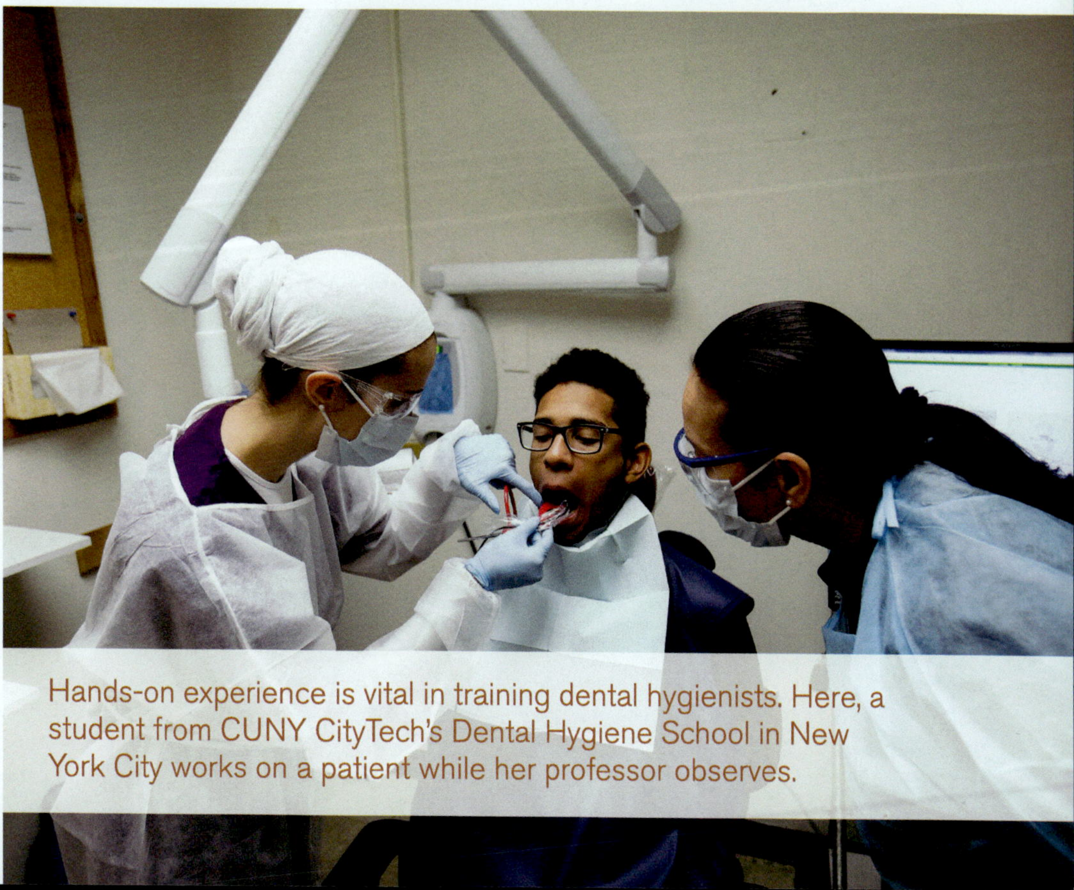

Hands-on experience is vital in training dental hygienists. Here, a student from CUNY CityTech's Dental Hygiene School in New York City works on a patient while her professor observes.

receive bachelor's and even master's degrees. These students often advance into research, public health, or educational health programs.

After receiving a diploma from a CODA-accredited program, the dental hygiene student must pass a rigorous written exam, the National Board Dental Hygiene Examination, followed by a state or regional clinical board examination. Only then does the student become a full-fledged registered dental hygienist, or RDH, and become able to practice. Continuing education keeps hygienists updated on current trends and furthers their knowledge in the field.

Dental hygienists are generally well paid. The median salary, according to a BLS report in October 2017, was $72,910 per year, or $35.05 per hour. Almost all hygienists worked in dentists' offices, and more than half worked part-time. The job outlook is excellent, with projected growth of 20 percent between 2016 and 2026. Most dental hygienists love their jobs and rate themselves "extremely satisfied," according to the website PayScale.com. Many remain dental hygienists for their entire careers. Those who obtain additional education may advance along several career paths. Some become registered nurses; others become office managers in dental offices. Both of these moves pay less than dental hygiene. Those who specialize in a field within dental hygiene (for example, periodontic dental hygiene) will see a salary increase. In all cases, dental hygiene is a respected and much-needed field that provides excellent job satisfaction for the right person.

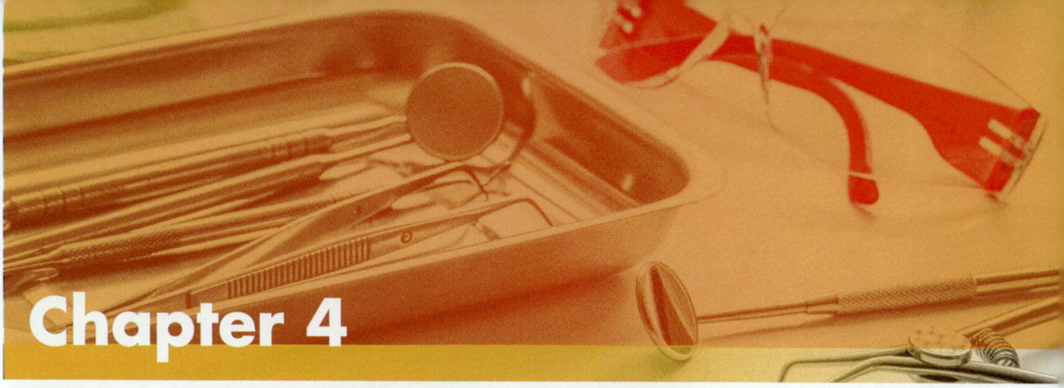

Chapter 4

EDUCATION FOR ALLIED DENTISTRY

Allied dental careers require much less training than the eight years of college and dental school required for a dentist. These fulfilling careers provide essential services for patients. Dental assistants, dental hygienists, and dental laboratory technicians are allied dental professionals who can complete training and be ready to practice in one to three years. Each field requires its own specific courses and training paths, but much of the preparation and education for the three fields is similar. For example, all allied dentistry students will benefit from taking STEM (science, technology, engineering, and math) courses in high school. The training programs themselves all include a combination of classroom, laboratory, and clinical experience. Coursework includes a strong grounding in science as well as training in techniques and technology geared toward each specific career.

What Courses Are Required?

A person considering an allied dentistry career can start preparing early by taking high school courses including health, biology, chemistry, psychology, mathematics, and speech. These courses are particularly important for students in dental hygiene or dental lab technology. Classes in shop and studio art, such as welding, carpentry, sculpture, ceramics, clay, and casting, can be beneficial for those who want to begin studies in dental lab technology. Hygienists tend to use more science knowledge, while lab technicians use more technology. However, both science and technology are valuable for the two fields. Dental assistants require less training in both areas. They are often responsible for office management work (such as maintaining patient files and managing appointments), making courses in business a plus. Nevertheless, a strong scientific and technological background will make the dental assistant a better employee and will make it easier for that person to advance in the field.

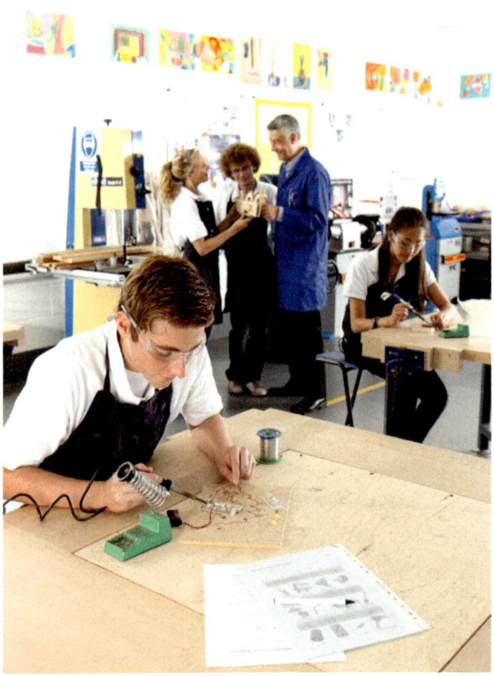

Shop-oriented classes in high school or vocational school prepare students before they attend allied dental school by giving them practice using small tools, such as soldering irons.

Those following the dental assistant career path can enroll with only a high school diploma. After a course lasting eight to twelve months, the graduate takes a certification exam and receives a certificate or diploma. Dental laboratory technicians (DLTs) can also enter a program directly from high school and can be fully qualified in two years. A few continue on to obtain four-year degrees. Dental hygiene programs often require applicants to complete at least one year of college before enrolling in the program. Those going for a bachelor's degree may need two years of college. College liberal arts courses, such as English, speech, sociology, and psychology, may be required as prerequisites for entering a dental hygiene program.

Dental assistant courses may include dental radiography (radiation safety and taking X-rays), dental anatomy and orthodontics, dental health (emphasizing periodontics, preventive dentistry, and nutrition), laboratory procedures (hands-on instruction in taking impressions and making casts), and dental specialties. The dental specialties course provides an overview of special skills needed in dental areas including implants, endodontics, periodontics, oral and maxillofacial surgery, and pedodontics (the study of children's teeth). Courses required for dental hygienists include anatomy, physiology, microbiology, immunology, dental hygiene, dental anatomy, radiology, periodontics, dental materials, pharmacology, patient pain management, nutrition, pathology, head and neck anatomy, and medical ethics.

DLTs must learn the structure of the mouth and how to make specific dental appliances. Their courses might include: dental anatomy and morphology, dental techniques, partial prosthodontics, materials for dental prosthetics, dental ceramics, and orthodontic appliance

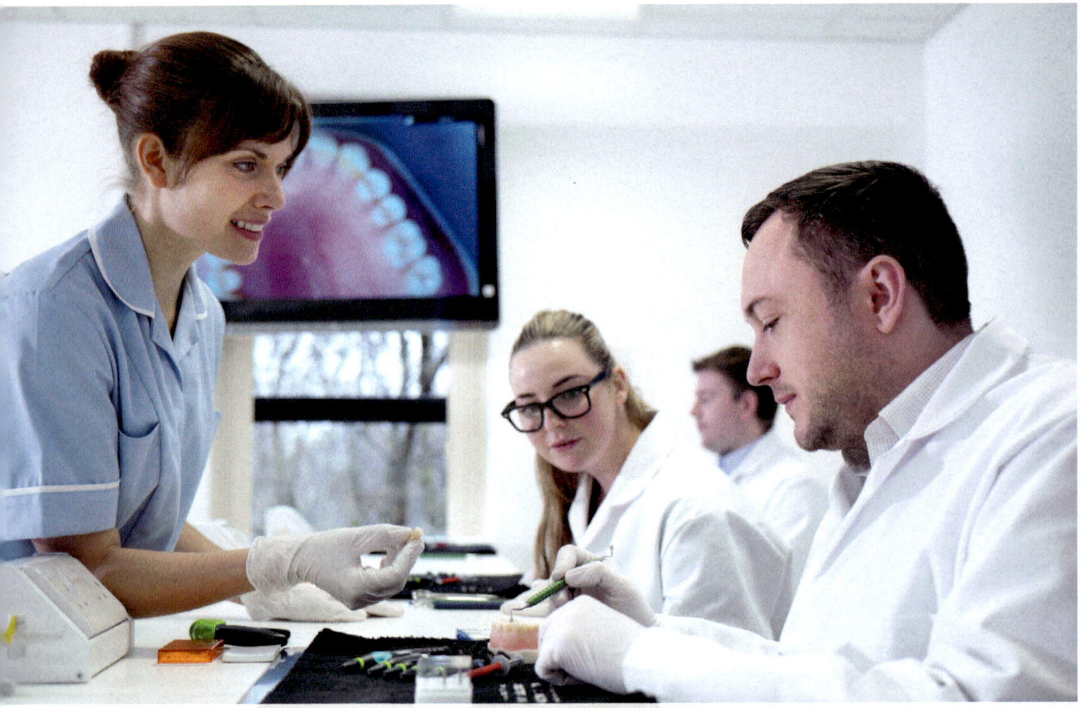

Before working on actual patients, allied dental trainees receive classroom training. They get their first hands-on experience by practicing the use of dental tools on mouth models.

construction. Gary Iocco is a former president of the National Association of Dental Laboratories. In an interview in 2017 with Fred Decker for Career Trend, Iocco advised aspiring DLTs to concentrate on the newest techniques, including 3D printing, scanning, designing, and milling. The field has shown little technological change for decades, but it is now exploding. "I think we're at the beginning of another golden age in dental laboratory technology," Iocco said.

Infection control is vital in the dental office, and an important part of allied dental certification exams. Dental practitioners are trained in infection control procedures, including sterilization of instruments and equipment and use of personal protective equipment. In 2003, the Centers for Disease Control and Prevention (CDC) published infection control guidelines for dentistry, which were updated in 2016. The CDC provides tools and resources to help dental offices comply with these guidelines and recommends periodic continuing education programs for every dental office. Additional resources are available from the Organization for Safety, Asepsis and Prevention (OSAP).

Online Learning

Some colleges and universities now offer online programs in dental assisting and dental hygiene. These encompass all coursework, including techniques such as sterilizing and preparing instruments. Many colleges now train dental assistants in four-handed dentistry, in which dental assistants work directly with dentists to complete clinical tasks more efficiently. Online programs prepare students to take state, regional, or national certification exams required to practice. Those considering online programs should ensure that the program is accredited. Most certification and licensure programs require graduation from an accredited program.

Online courses are excellent for students who need flexibility. These include people who have family or work obligations or who live far from the nearest training program. Many online programs are self-paced; students can take as much or as little time as they need to complete them, and they can study anytime, anywhere. Programs vary; for example, the US Career Institute allows dental assisting students to choose from a standard program or an enhanced program that includes supplements and additional tools. Online courses also provide continuing education courses required to maintain a license in allied dental fields.

The website BestColleges.com listed the five best colleges for 2018 for providing online dental assistant training. They are the following: Indiana University-Purdue University-Indianapolis (IUPUI, Indianapolis, Indiana), Oregon State University (OSU, Corvallis, Oregon), Rutgers University (New Brunswick, New Jersey), Ozarks Technical Community College (OTC, Springfield, Missouri), and Monroe Community College (MCC, Monroe County, New York).

Students in the IUPUI program complete all nonclinical coursework online. They travel to campus one or two Saturdays per month to complete pre-clinical work, labs, and exams. After graduating, they are eligible to take the DANB exam.

The OSU program is done online with faculty and student mentors. OSU recommends, but does not require, a clinical externship. Full-time students usually complete the course in six months.

Rutgers offers an administrative dental assistant certificate program, which can be completed in six months. This completely online course concentrates on the office management aspects of dental assisting, such as medical records, diagnostic coding, and billing and insurance.

OTC's program is CODA-accredited and leads to state and national credentials. It emphasizes dental anatomy, materials, and equipment; chairside assisting; infection control; and radiology. All nonclinical coursework is done online. Labs, clinical instruction, and clinical rotations are done on Saturdays on campus.

MCC's coursework is similar to OTC's and leads to licensure in two semesters. There is no internship or campus attendance; instead, employers provide on-the-job clinical training.

Practical Considerations

Aspiring allied dental health students might begin by researching the fields online. Once students have a good idea of which field meets their needs, they can look for specific programs and rank them according to location, cost, and other factors unique to each student's situation.

One important factor is financial aid. The American Dental Association Foundation (ADAF) operates a scholarship program, the Allied Dental Student Scholarship. Every year, they award fifteen scholarships in dental hygiene, ten in dental assistance, and five in dental laboratory technology. The National Dental Association Foundation Colgate-Palmolive Scholarship offers aid to underrepresented minority students around the country. Federally funded scholarships include Scholarships for Disadvantaged Students, the National Health Service Corps (NHSC), Armed Forces Health Professions Scholarship, and others. Some branches of the military offer financial aid or loan forgiveness in exchange for a work commitment. National student loans are also

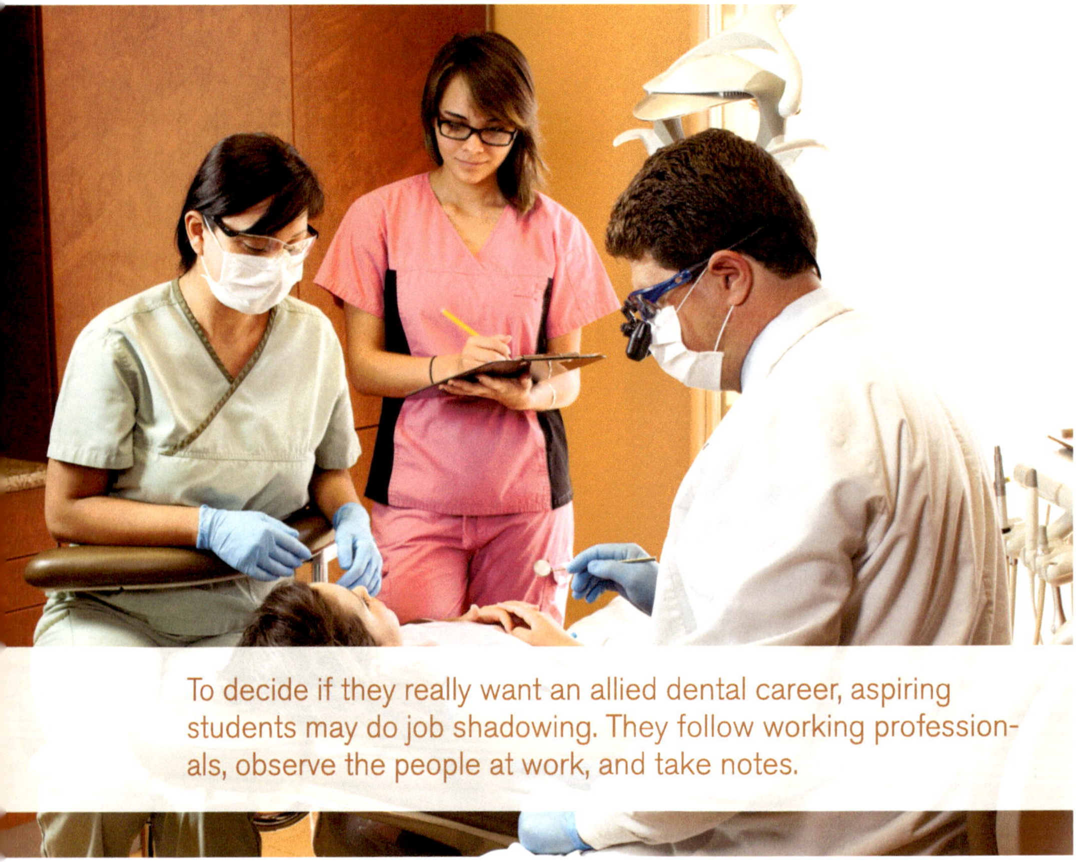

To decide if they really want an allied dental career, aspiring students may do job shadowing. They follow working professionals, observe the people at work, and take notes.

available. Work-study programs are often available at each school. Students should contact the school they plan to attend and ask about financial aid.

To become proficient in any field, on-the-job experience is essential. For allied dental fields, this practical knowledge often includes internships or externships that provide hands-on work experience. Usually, the intern (or extern) participates in simple jobs and learns new skills. Tiffany Kurzawa is associate director at the Center for

JOB SHADOWING

Job shadowing is an excellent way to find out exactly what is required in an allied dental job. Some programs require it and may assist their students in finding a person to shadow. Other schools prefer that students job-shadow before enrolling. To find an allied dental professional to shadow, the first stop is a person's own dental office. Ask the dental assistant or hygienist if they are willing to be shadowed or if they can recommend someone else. Ask friends, classmates, parents, and others. When you locate someone to shadow, communicate clearly with that person. Set a time and be punctual. Dress professionally and comfortably—you will spend the day on your feet, so do not wear high heels. Learn the names of all office staff members, not just the one you are shadowing, and be friendly. Ask questions and take notes. Possible questions include: What do you like most about your job? What is most challenging? If you could do it over, would you still choose this career? What advice do you have for me?

Career Development at Gettysburg College. According to Kurzawa (quoted by Jacquelyn Smith in *Forbes*), "Externships are valuable career learning experiences in that they provide the opportunity for students to see first-hand what the day-to-day work activities and responsibilities are."

After completing the educational part of allied dental school, the final step is certification, obtained by passing an intensive exam process. There is a required certification exam (or several) in each allied dentistry field. Usually, there are separate exams—a comprehensive written exam and at least one exam that tests hands-on skills and clinical knowledge. For example,

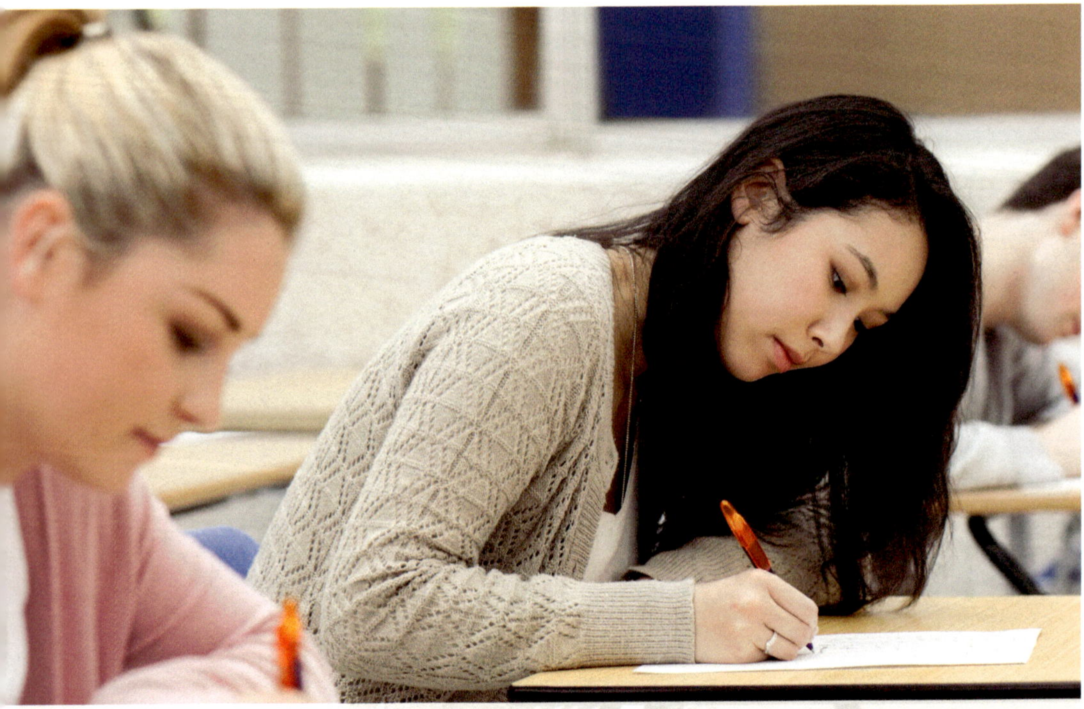

Although probably not the most fun, one required part of training for an allied dental career is taking an extensive series of exams, both written and practical.

prospective dental assistants take the Certified Dental Assistant (CDA) exam, from the DANB. The CDA exam takes four hours and consists of 320 questions in three sections: general chairside test (120 questions), radiation health and safety (100 questions), and infection control test (100 questions).

A student who has graduated from an accredited school and passed all required licensing exams is fully qualified to obtain employment as an allied dental health professional.

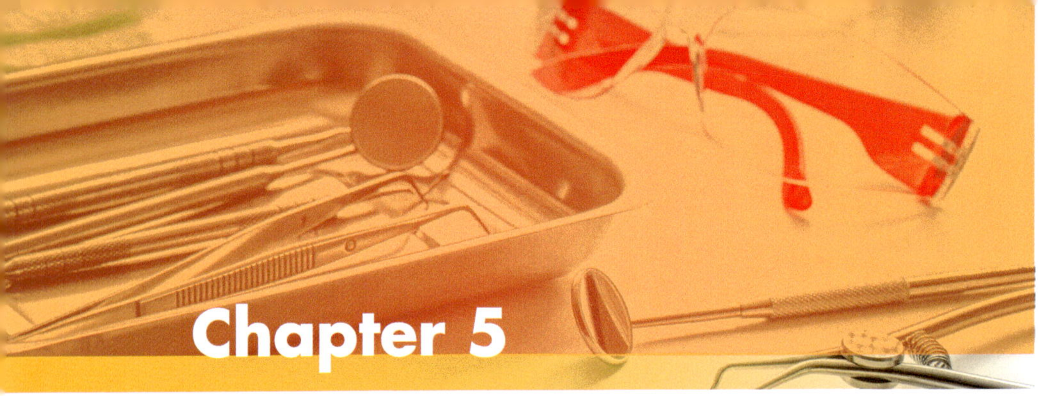

Chapter 5

FINDING A JOB IN ALLIED DENTISTRY

Students have completed an accredited program in allied dentistry. They passed their licensure exams with flying colors. These former hard-working students are now fully licensed dental assistants, dental hygienists, or dental lab technicians—and are ready for their first professional jobs. Now they have a new set of hurdles: Where to look? What to look for? How to apply? How to interview? What to do on the first day?

Looking for a Job

Dental programs the students attended, their guidance counselors, and people in their employment offices know the field and maintain job listings for companies and offices in the area. The ADA has an online career center that allows job seekers to search for jobs by job type and state. Other possibilities are job centers, employment offices, job fairs, or career websites such as Indeed.com and Monster.com. Online health care staffing agencies, such as HealthPro Staffing Resources, provide employment opportunities in the dental field and can help place job seekers in temporary or permanent positions, many of which offer flexible schedules.

Doug and Tracie Perry, authors of the book *Landing a Great Dental Hygiene Job*, concentrate on dental hygienists, but their suggestions apply equally well to dental assistants or dental lab technicians. The Perrys suggest that, to make applications stand out, job applicants should prepare a marketing package consisting of four documents: résumé, cover letter, testimonial sheet, and a challenge-action-resolution (CAR) sheet.

A résumé for a clinical job in a dentist's office should be one page in length and should follow a functional format. After the heading (which includes the name, contact information, and a brief description of the applicant), it should have short sections listing the applicant's experience and skills; work history, including apprenticeships; education history; and (space permitting)

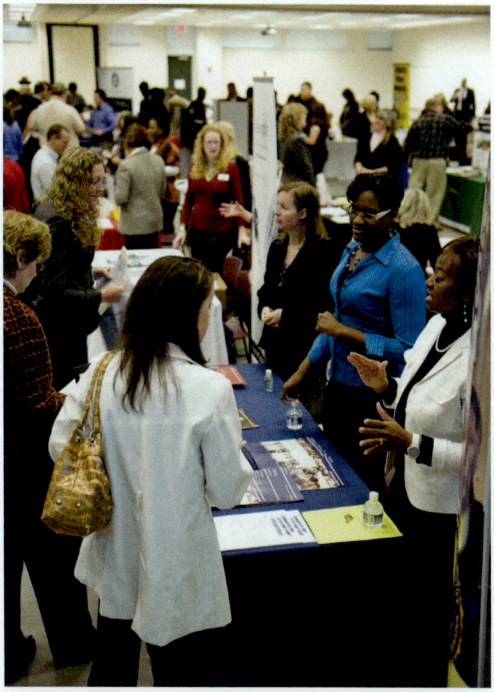

After completing coursework, certification, and exams, the allied dental professional must find a job. Local and university job fairs enable job seekers to talk with people from hiring companies.

association memberships, licenses, community service, and other relevant information. A cover letter is vital. It allows applicants to summarize their qualifications for each specific job. It should address how the applicant meets each qualification in the job listing. It makes the application more personal and distinguishes the applicant from others. It should end with a call to action, asking for an interview and giving directions for reaching the applicant.

Doug and Tracie Perry describe the testimonial sheet as "third-party validation of the claims you make about yourself." It contains three to five short quotations from employers, teachers, or past clients, describing the applicant's best skills and qualities. The applicant should always obtain permission to use quotations. Ideally, quotations should come from reference letters. The CAR sheet is a short list of mini case studies. These are examples of problems applicants have faced with patients (challenge), how the applicant handled them (action), and how the situation turned out (resolution). This material shows the potential employer that the applicant can successfully overcome problems or crises in the workplace. Developing the testimonial sheets and CAR sheets is extra work for applicants, but that is the point. They make an applicant stand out and demonstrate a good attitude and a strong work ethic.

Although the outlook for allied dental jobs is good, job seekers will not always land their dream job on the first try. This situation is especially true in a saturated market, such as an area with one or more large allied dental programs. It may be necessary to take whatever job comes along, including a part-time job. It is always easier to obtain a new job if you already have one, and every job teaches new skills that will make the applicant more marketable next time. Also, the more licenses new dental professionals have, the more appealing they will be to prospective employers. A dental hygienist who is qualified to administer local anesthetics will be more valuable than one who is not.

Surviving the Interview

Tija Hunter, a dental assistant and office manager for thirty years, is in charge of hiring at her dental office. In an article on DentistryIQ.com, she summed up the challenge of hiring: "I can teach anyone to be a dental

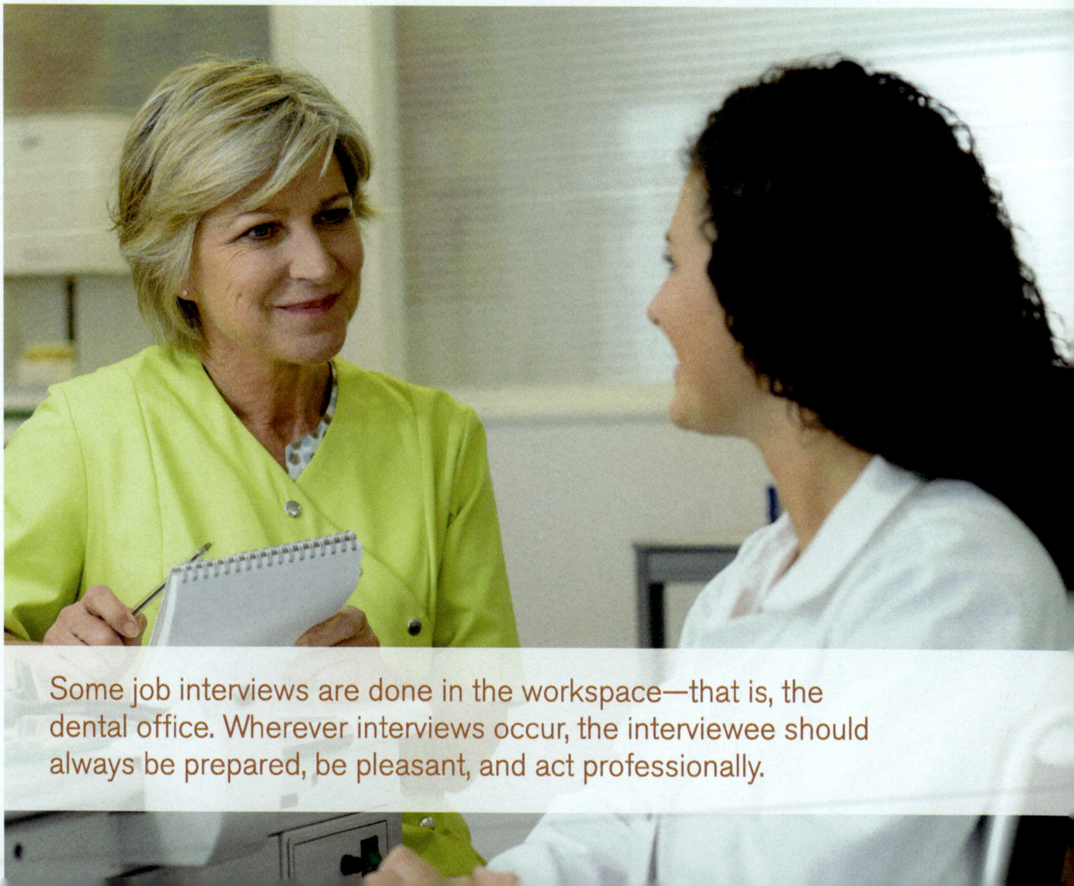

Some job interviews are done in the workspace—that is, the dental office. Wherever interviews occur, the interviewee should always be prepared, be pleasant, and act professionally.

assistant ... yes, anyone. What I can't teach is attitude." Hunter wants to hire a hard worker with eagerness and enthusiasm for the job. She gives some guidelines for the application process: when dropping off an application or attending an interview, make a good first impression. Don't smoke or chew gum; dress neatly and professionally and make sure you comb your hair; speak professionally and use proper grammar. Don't email or fax your résumé; deliver it personally. Smile, make eye contact, chat with the office staff, and be specific about the purpose of your visit. If you must email or fax an application, definitely include an outstanding cover letter.

Interviewees should bring extra copies of their marketing package (including proof of certification) to the interview, along with contact information for three to five references. They should arrive no more than ten minutes early, introduce themselves to the receptionist, and be friendly. When speaking during the interview, they should avoid nervous fillers such as "um," "like," and "you know," and instead, pause and gather their thoughts before speaking. Interviewees should talk no more than one-third of the time. They should listen carefully and respond to the interviewer with good comments or questions. They should refer to the position in the third person, rather than acting as though the job is theirs. For example, say "Does the dental hygienist schedule return appointments?" rather than "Will I be scheduling return appointments?" When appropriate, interviewees should sell themselves, inserting comments (prepared and rehearsed in advance) detailing their best qualifications for the job.

COMMON INTERVIEW QUESTIONS

Considering interview questions and possible answers in advance is one way to prepare for an interview. Even for general questions, good answers will relate to the specific job. Answering the question "Tell me about yourself" might involve a brief statement of career objectives, as well as comments about family, education, and previous jobs. An answer to "What are your strengths and weaknesses?" should discuss both in relation to the job. Interviewees should also prepare short but thoughtful responses to specific questions, for example: Why does the dental field interest you? What are your long-term career goals, and how will being a dental assistant (or hygienist or lab tech) help you meet them? What do you consider the most valuable skill for a dental assistant (or hygienist or lab tech)? How would you handle a situation where a patient is not satisfied? When asked, "What questions do you have for me?" the interviewee's questions should show that he or she has researched the company and wants to contribute to it.

According to RDHmag.com, registered dental hygienist Eva M. Watson takes a pen

(continued on the next page)

(continued from the previous page)

and notebook to interviews and asks permission to ask questions and take notes. She asks questions such as: How many active patients does the practice have? How much treatment time is allotted for each hygiene patient? Is marketing money available for the practice? Other dental professionals suggest these questions: What is your policy for replacing dental instruments? Can I review the employee manual before accepting the position? Do you provide a stipend for continuing education or a professional discount for dental treatment? Questions asked will vary, but organized interviewees always research the company and come prepared with intelligent questions.

Interviewees should always ask questions. Good questions to ask early in the interview are "What characteristics do you most want in the person you hire?" or "What are your most important priorities for this job?" Thereafter, they can tailor their responses to answer these questions. Later in the interview, asking questions such as "Do you have any concerns about my abilities or qualifications?" will provide an opportunity to counter an interviewer's possible concerns. Salary should only be discussed if the interviewer brings it up; it is negotiated after the job is offered. Sometimes interviewers ask odd or even illegal questions to test the interviewee. Deciding in advance how to field such questions can show interviewees' ability to think on their feet and recover. Immediately after every interview, send the interviewer a short thank-you note.

The First Days of Work

Careful preparation can decrease the stress of starting a new job. Preparation begins at the interview, by finding out as much as possible about the dental office, how busy it is, and exactly what is expected of the new employee. On RDHmag.com, Kara Vavrosky, a registered dental hygienist, shared five tips that a new employee should keep in mind—not only on the first day, but at least the first one hundred days—to make it easier to integrate into a new job situation. First, always put patients first. Begin immediately to develop a rapport with them. Learn to communicate and listen to their concerns. Second, be organized. Learn where everything is and develop a system that works for you. Third, show yourself to be a team player by going above and beyond your duties. Take out the trash, restock supplies—in short, do whatever is needed. Fourth, learn office culture so you can fit in. Learn the hierarchy and how things are done. Finally, be enthusiastic and don't be discouraged when things don't go well. Every job has ups and downs and becomes easier with time and experience.

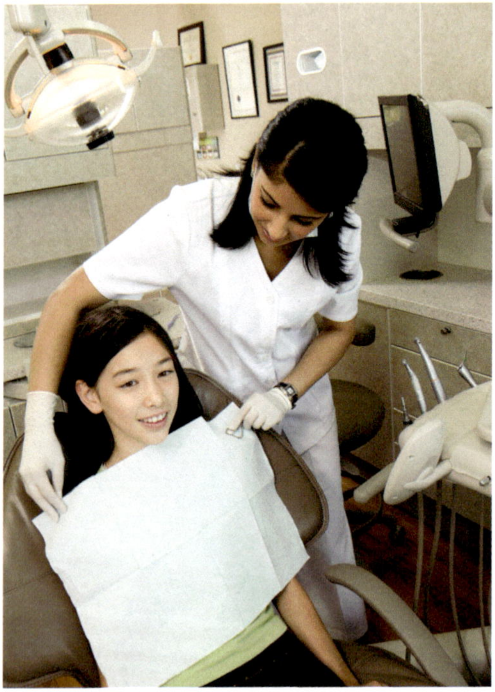

All new dental assistants or hygienists undergo a learning curve in a new job, but one thing they can always do is be friendly and make their patients comfortable.

One thing many new dental professionals overlook is the physical toll the job takes. When an employee is busy and on one's feet for hours on end, fatigue becomes a real problem. Dental professionals must take care of their own physical and mental health and develop and practice fatigue-reducing strategies. Finally, remember that becoming a professional takes time and practice. Learning does not stop when school is over. It continues on the job and requires constant updating of clinical skills through continuing education.

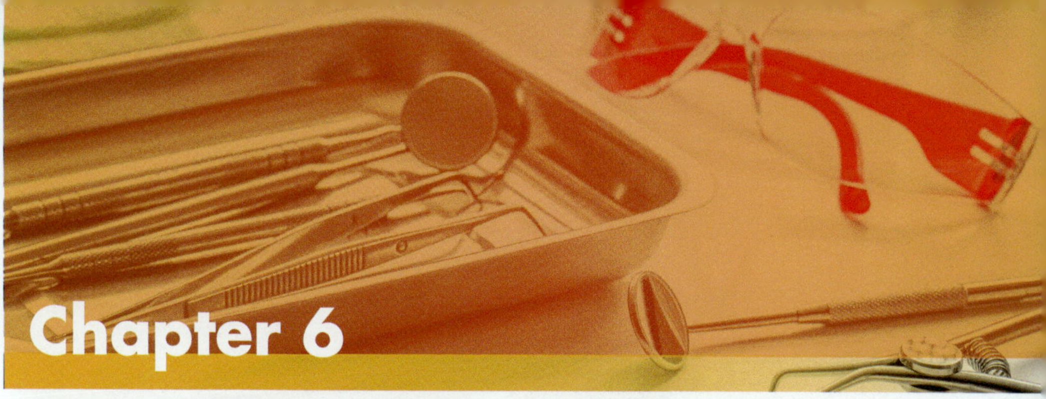

Chapter 6

STRATEGIES FOR SUCCESS IN ALLIED DENTISTRY

Beyond the first one hundred days, what can allied dentistry professionals do to excel in the workplace? How can they ensure that their careers progress and improve? Three sure ways to succeed include developing good work habits, constantly learning on the job, and staying up to date through continuing education.

Work Habits

The number one goal for the dental assistant or hygienist is to serve the patient and the dentist. Thus, success in both fields requires a love of assisting and a desire to serve. Being of service entails respect, compassion, and empathy. Excellent assistants or hygienists understand the patients' fear or nervousness and allay their fears by listening well, showing respect and consideration, and communicating the information the patients need. The goal of service requires a warm, friendly personality, but it also requires the assistant to be intelligent and well informed in the field. A good sense of humor helps, too.

Making patients laugh or see the humor in a situation can ease their nervousness.

An integral part of being an excellent dental assistant or hygienist is being well organized and well prepared for each day's work. For example, dental assistants, as the link between patient and dentist, must show professionalism at all times and do it with a smile and a friendly attitude. They do their best to make sure procedures flow smoothly, with as little discomfort to the patient as possible. Being detail-oriented and thorough in your preparations, procedures, and cleanup will help make you an excellent (not just a good) dental professional.

In addition to patients, dental assistants and hygienists must work seamlessly with office staff members—other hygienists and assistants as well as the dentist. One characteristic that will help a good dental professional become an excellent one is integrity. A person with integrity always tries to do the right thing. Another is good teamwork. Being a team player means working well with other staff members—doing necessary chores without complaint, offering to help when someone is struggling or has a heavy workload, and generally being pleasant to be around. Always striving to learn and improve oneself is another valuable characteristic. This supplemental education might mean on-the-job training or taking courses to learn new skills and techniques. More and better skills make for a more valuable employee.

Like all new employees, DLTs should immediately learn their workspace and the location of all items and always keep their workstations impeccably clean and neat. They should ask a lot of questions and develop a routine that fits with other team members and promotes a smooth

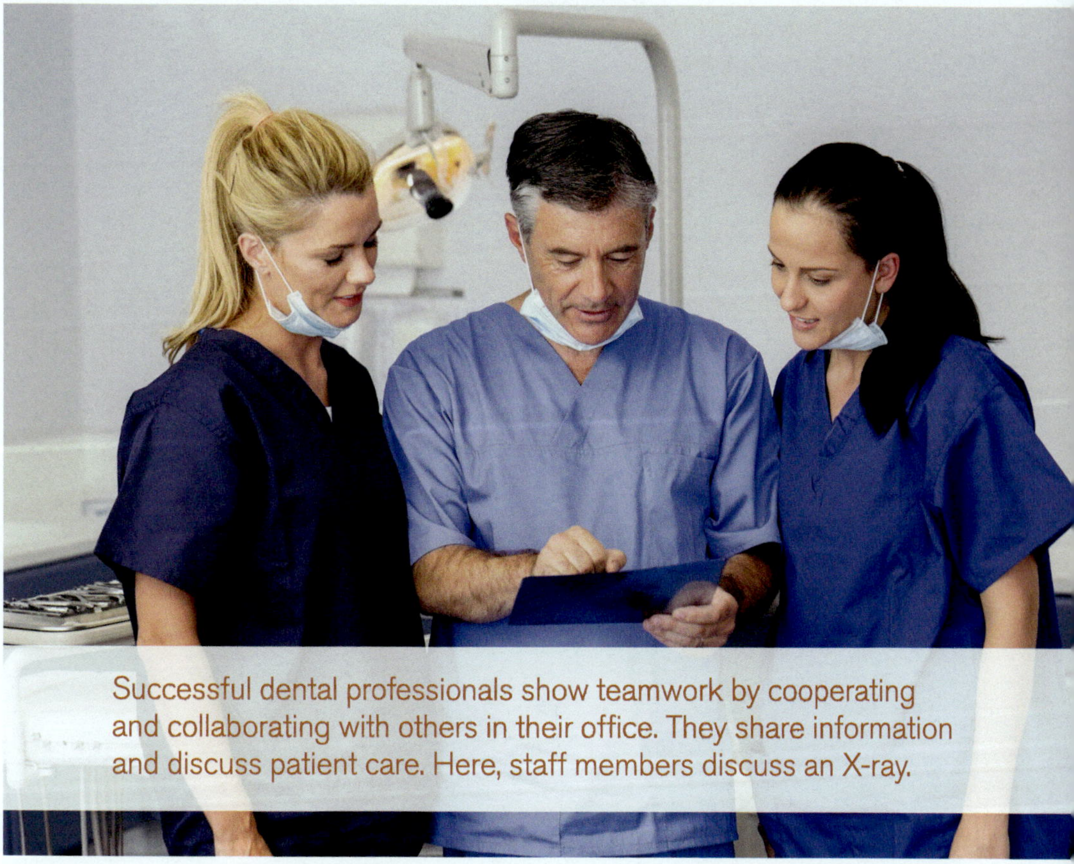

Successful dental professionals show teamwork by cooperating and collaborating with others in their office. They share information and discuss patient care. Here, staff members discuss an X-ray.

workflow. This regimen includes figuring out the approximate time it takes to finish each task, so work can be planned, scheduled, and completed on time. Self-motivation is perhaps more valuable for DLTs than other allied dental professionals, because the work does not involve a constant flow of patients. Although people skills are perhaps less valued because DLTs do not see patients, they are still important. Befriending colleagues and being a kind and thoughtful labmate will result in a friendlier workplace and make the DLT an appreciated team member.

Dental laboratory technicians should also work constantly to perfect the skills essential in their field, including attention to detail, hand-eye coordination, and color perception. Because each dental patient is unique, these skills must be developed to ensure that each patient receives a dental appliance that is precisely suited in color and fit. DLTs can also improve their lab skills through personal activities. For example, DLTs who create art as a hobby can improve their artistic skills and color perception. They can improve hand-eye coordination by playing musical instruments, video games, or certain sports.

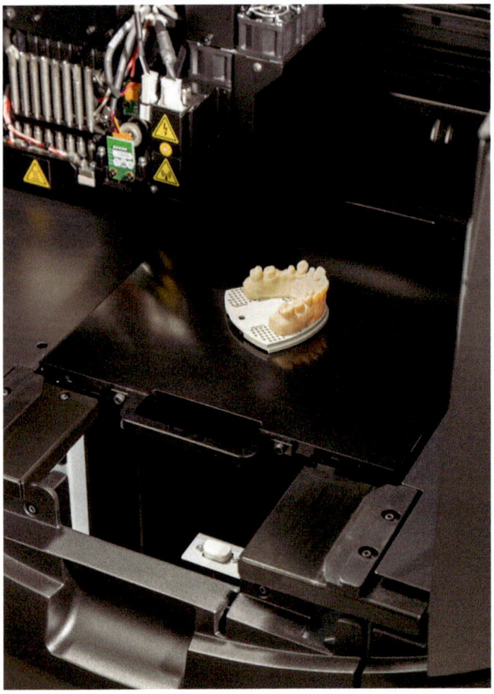

This 3D printer has just printed a dental implant bridge. Dental lab technicians can advance their careers by keeping up to date on new equipment and technology.

On-the-Job Training

At least in the beginning, most of an allied dental professional's development will occur through on-the-job training. This training involves getting used to the routine and learning the quirks of the job—what is expected and where the new employee fits in. New employees should be observant, quickly learning where equipment and supplies are located and how things are done. They should always be willing to ask questions of other employees. They should keep up to date by seeking out current information. These particularly include informative websites such as DentistryIQ.com and the websites of professional associations—American Dental Assistants Association (ADAA), American Dental Hygienists Association (ADHA), or National Association of Dental Laboratories (NADL). Participation in local or state

THE IMPORTANCE OF MENTORS

Mentors are guides who teach by example, helping mentees build and expand their own skills. They set an example that mentees can follow and imitate. They share experiences and answer questions. Good mentors believe in their mentees and demand excellence from them. They provide mentees with opportunities to prove themselves. New dental assistants or hygienists may encounter difficult patients or situations and be unsure what to do. A mentor who has been through similar experiences can provide advice and reassurance. Anyone with knowledge and expertise can be a mentor. One multigenerational dental office practiced mentorship across the

(continued on the next page)

(continued from the previous page)

generations. The older front-desk administrator, struggling with new computer software, asked the generation-X dental assistant to teach her. A millennial hygienist encountered a worrying wound on a young patient's chin, which the patient refused to explain. She consulted the baby-boomer hygienist, who volunteered at a women's clinic, and watched in awe as the older woman got the young patient to open up. A close mentor-mentee relationship between two people is valuable, but for the observant dental employee, anyone around them can become a mentor.

chapters of these organizations allows interaction with other professionals, which provides both support and lifelong learning.

Ideally, career development also involves finding a mentor who can answer questions, teach new skills, give advice on how to handle certain patients or situations, and generally provide support. Mentors do not have to be older, just more experienced. They do not have to be in the same office (although that is convenient) or even in the same field, if the problem is general (for example, dealing with difficult people). Good mentors can be located by consulting past classmates or teachers; websites, clubs, or panels in the field; professional associations; or obtaining referrals from others in the field. Good mentors might provide reference materials to read, offer advice or constructive criticism (which should be taken graciously and considered seriously), or suggest sources for continuing education.

Lifelong Learning

Becoming and remaining a valuable dental professional always involves lifelong learning. Continuing education is necessary to stay informed in any career, especially allied dental fields. Continuing education credits are available for dental assistants, hygienists, and lab techs. These courses can be found through local or regional sources, such as schools and colleges offering allied dental

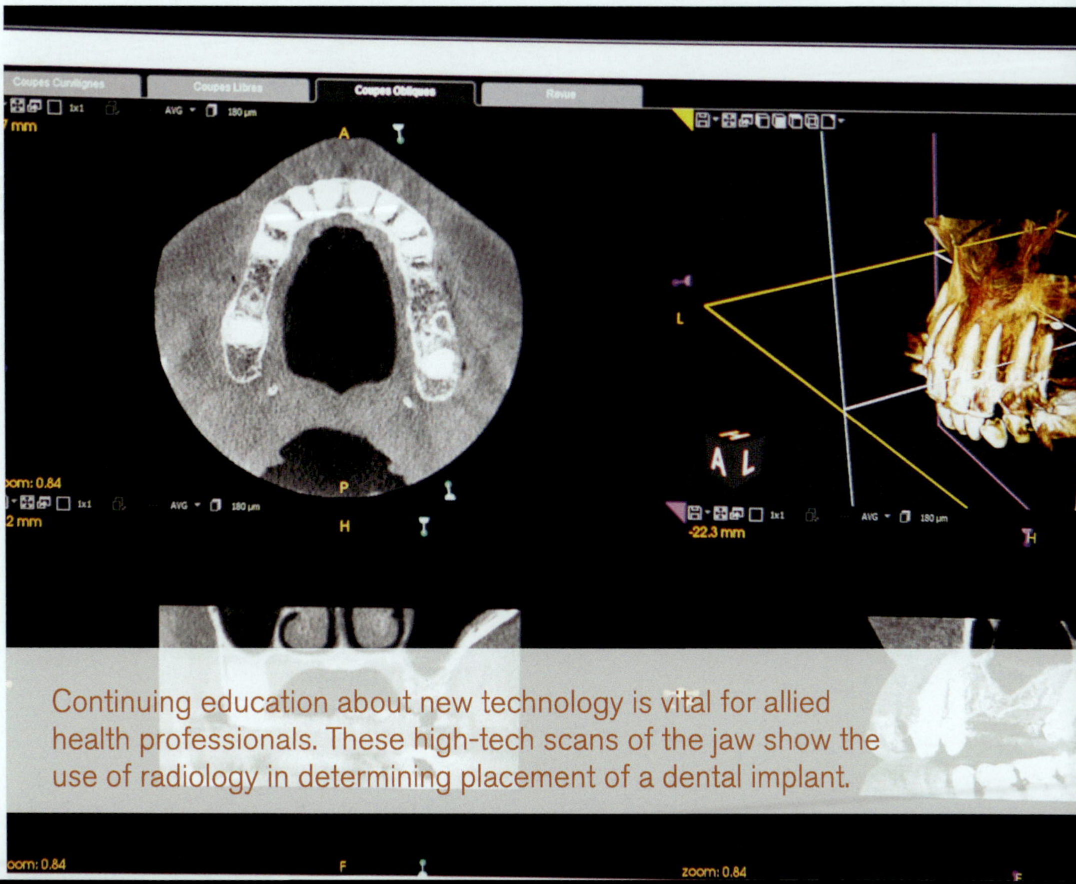

Continuing education about new technology is vital for allied health professionals. These high-tech scans of the jaw show the use of radiology in determining placement of a dental implant.

degrees. There are also many online resources. The professional organizations for all three allied dental jobs (ADAA, ADHA, and NADL) offer continuing education courses and webinars online. The website dentalcare.com, run by Proctor & Gamble (Crest and OralB), and Colgate's Oral Health Network offer free continuing education courses and webinars for dental assistants and dental hygienists.

For DLTs who want to advance, particularly to start their own businesses, continuing education is extremely valuable. DLTs should attain additional specialties, as well as take business courses. An especially valuable skill is having an understanding of CAD/CAM technology. This

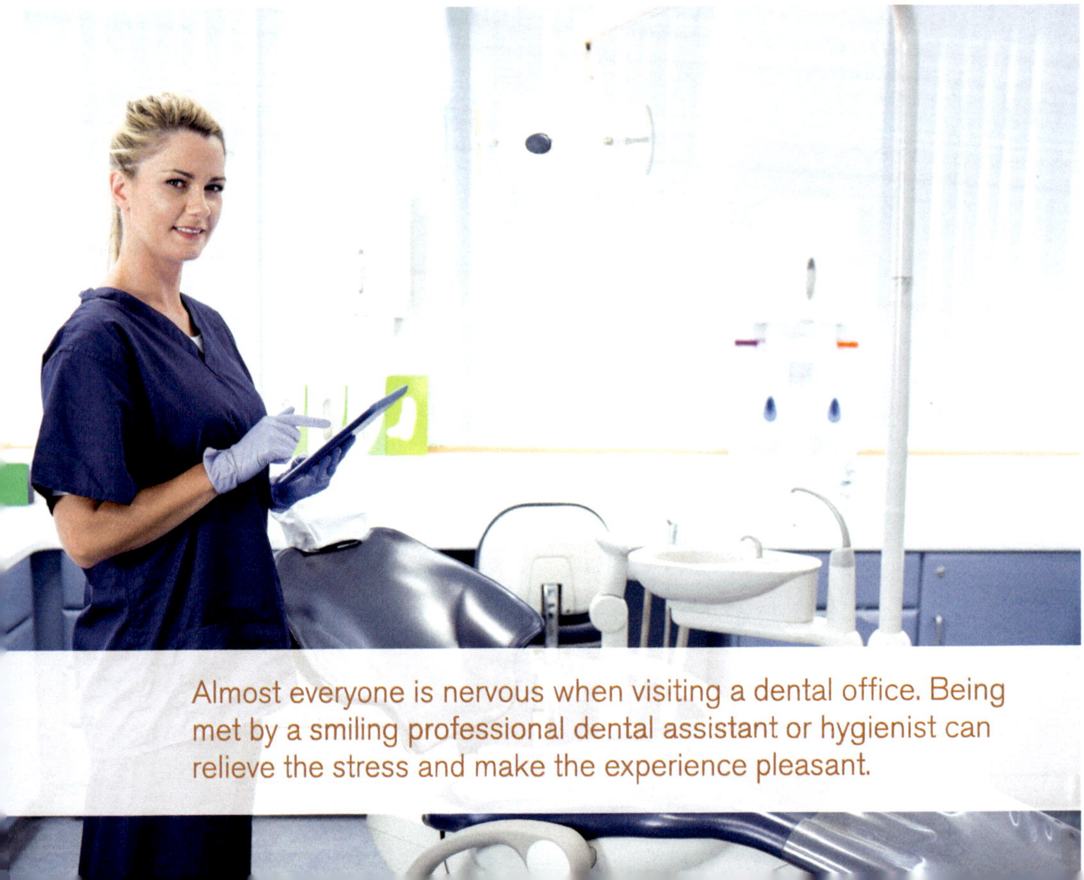

Almost everyone is nervous when visiting a dental office. Being met by a smiling professional dental assistant or hygienist can relieve the stress and make the experience pleasant.

knowledge should be mastered by every DLT who aspires to excellence. CAD is computer-assisted design, and CAM is computer-assisted manufacturing. CAD/CAM software enables DLTs to work with digital 3D models of the patient's teeth, rather than making physical impressions and molds. CAD/CAM is fast, precise, and uses cutting-edge materials. But equipment and software are expensive, and technicians must be trained. A DLT trained in CAD/CAM procedures will be an essential employee.

The allied dental professions are growing career areas that can provide steady, meaningful employment for people interested in dental health. They are relatively easy to enter, requiring as little as a year of training (or even, in some cases, only a high school diploma and on-the-job training). All three fields provide opportunities for advancement if employees keep their skills sharp and constantly improve their knowledge through continuing education. These careers are not for everyone, so aspiring dental professionals should carefully consider whether they would enjoy the work and find it satisfying. They should ask themselves, "Would I enjoy coming to work every morning? Would I enjoy helping people maintain healthy teeth and smiles, and would I be good at it?" If the answer to these questions is yes, then a career in dental assisting, dental hygiene, or dental lab technology may be a great choice for you.

GLOSSARY

accredited Officially recognized and authorized by an agency or organization; for example, an accredited dental assistant program.

allied dentistry professions Dental professionals who work with and assist dentists but have less training; these include dental assistants, hygienists, and lab technicians.

bridge A fixed dental structure that replaces one or more missing teeth by anchoring the fixed replacement to adjacent teeth on either side.

carpal tunnel syndrome A condition that can cause tingling, numbness, and weakness in a hand or arm. It is caused by pressure on a nerve in the carpal tunnel, a narrow passageway on the palm side of the wrist.

certification A formal certificate or other credential bestowed after a person has completed education and training and has passed one or more exams given by a professional licensing authority; often required before a person can be hired as an allied dentistry professional.

cover letter A letter written to accompany a résumé; it introduces the job applicant and describes the applicant's specific skills and qualifications for the job in question.

crown A cap or covering on a tooth that restores it to its original size and shape; often bonded to the tooth using dental cement, it is used to restore teeth with large cavities.

dental assistant An allied dental professional who assists dentists in whatever ways are needed, from making patients comfortable to office work to cleanup; some do special procedures such as taking X-rays.

dental hygienist An allied dental professional who is trained to clean teeth by removing plaque and tartar and to generally maintain tooth health by doing visual inspections of teeth, applying sealants and fluorides, and educating patients on home dental care.

dental laboratory technician An allied dental professional who is trained to mold and construct dental appliances, such as night guards, braces, dentures, bridges, and crowns; he or she works in a laboratory and has little contact with patients.

dentures A set of artificial teeth used to replace teeth lost through decay, disease, or accident; dentures can be full (replacing all teeth) or partial (replacing only a portion of the teeth).

externship A training program made available by a university or private company or medical office, offering a student a short-term (usually unpaid) practical work experience in that individual's field of study; it is similar to an internship or apprenticeship.

job shadowing Learning about the day-to-day activities involved in a job by following (shadowing) a person doing that job (a dental hygiene student would shadow a practicing dental hygienist).

mentor A person who serves as a close, but informal, teacher who helps a new employee by answering questions, teaching new skills, giving advice, and otherwise helping the employee adjust to a new career.

morphology In biology, the field that deals with the form and structure of animals and plants.

orthodontist A dentist who specializes in the prevention or correction of irregular teeth, usually by use of braces; the branch of dentistry is known as orthodontics.

pedodontics The branch of dentistry dealing with children's teeth.

periodontal Referring to the gums or other tissues encircling the teeth; for instance, periodontal disease is gum disease.

personal protective equipment (PPE) Equipment that includes a plastic barrier jacket and bonnet, a face mask, a face shield or eye protection, surgical gloves, and booties; all maintain clean surgical conditions to prevent infection during the work of dental hygienists and other medical or dental professionals.

plaque A sticky film of bacteria growing on teeth. It builds up when teeth are not brushed and collects between teeth and under gums; bacterial acids break down enamel and cause tooth decay.

practicum A practical section of a course of study, in which students practice the skills they have learned under supervision.

prosthodontics Restorative dentistry, or creation of dental appliances such as bridges, crowns, or dentures to return normal fit and function; used to replace teeth lost to decay, disease, illness, or accident.

radiology The science that uses medical imaging (such as X-rays) to diagnose and sometimes treat diseases, including diseases of the teeth; because it involves radiation, those using radiology must have special safety training.

résumé A formal, one-page summary of a job applicant's credentials; it includes sections for experience and skills, work history, education, and (if space permits) other related material such as internships and professional memberships.

retainer The part of a dental appliance (such as a bridge or brace) used to hold the appliance in place within the mouth; for example, the part of a bridge that attaches it to adjoining teeth.

tartar (also called dental calculus) A buildup of plaque on the teeth that has hardened or mineralized; it is harder to remove than plaque and must be removed by scaling and polishing.

ultrasonic scaler An instrument with a tip that uses ultrasonic vibrations (higher than the wavelengths that humans can hear) to loosen and remove deposits (plaque and tartar) from teeth.

FOR MORE INFORMATION

All Allied Health Schools
All Star Directories, Inc.
101 Stewart Street, Suite 500
Seattle, WA 98101
(877) 222-8251
Website: https://www.allalliedhealthschools.com
Facebook: @All Allied Health Schools
Instagram and Twitter: @AlliedHealthed
This organization's website is an online directory of accredited colleges and universities with degrees in the various healthcare fields. Students can search for programs by location, degree, and type.

American Dental Assistants Association (ADAA)
140 North Bloomingdale Road
Bloomingdale, IL 60108-1017
(877) 874-3785
Website: https://www.adaausa.org
Facebook: @adaa247
The website for the professional organization of dental assistants encourages and supports those in dental assisting careers through instruction and learning, laws and regulations, obtaining the appropriate credentials, and various professional programs.

American Dental Association (ADA)
211 East Chicago Avenue
Chicago, IL 60611-2678
(312) 440-2500
Website: http://www.ada.org/en
Facebook: @AmericanDentalAssociation
Instagram and Twitter: @AmerDentalAssn

The ADA is the professional organization for dentists and the leading source of dental health information for dentists and patients. The website includes information on continuing education and the ADA's publications. The ADA is a nonprofit organization.

American Dental Education Association (ADEA)
655 K Street NW, Suite 800
Washington, DC 20001
(202) 289-7201
Website: http://www.adea.org
Facebook: @ADEAweb
Instagram and Twitter: @adeaweb
The ADEA is the only national organization representing dental education. Its members include students, faculty, and staff of dental and allied dental schools. They determine best practices and advocate for public policy in dental education.

American Dental Hygienists' Association (ADHA)
444 North Michigan Avenue, Suite 400
Chicago, IL 60611
(312) 440-8900
Website: https://www.adha.org
Facebook: @youradha
Instagram and Twitter: @YourADHA
The ADHA represents dental hygienists around the United States. It provides training, educational information, and news updates regarding the dental hygienist field. It also develops additional career pathways and helps to support advancement for dental hygienists and comprehensive dental care.

Bureau of Labor Statistics (BLS)
US Department of Labor
2 Massachusetts Avenue NE, Suite 2135
Washington, DC 20212-0001
(202) 691-5700
Web site: http://www.bls.gov
This federal agency analyzes the labor market activity, industry working environments, and price changes in the US economy. Annually, the BLS updates the *Occupational Outlook Handbook* (https://www.bls.gov/ooh), which outlines thousands of careers and presents specifics about job requirements and average salaries.

Canadian Dental Association (CDA)
1815 Alta Vista Drive
Ottawa, ON K1G 3Y6
Canada
(613) 523-1770
Website: https://www.cda-adc.ca/en/index.asp
Facebook: @CanadianDentalAssociation
Instagram and Twitter: @CdnDentalAssoc
The CDA is the national organization representing Canadian dentists. It works to promote optimal oral health and to advance the profession.

Canadian Dental Hygienists Association (CDHA)
1122 Wellington Street W
Ottawa, ON K1Y 2Y7
Canada
(800) 267-5235
Website: http://www.cdha.ca

Facebook, Instagram, and Twitter: @theCDHA
The CDHA seeks to support Canadian dental hygienists through sharing of professional knowledge and research and promoting public policy that allows members to practice independently and inter-professionally.

Dentistry IQ–The Web's Most Comprehensive Resource for Dental Professionals
1421 South Sheridan Road
Tulsa, OK 74112
(800) 331-4463
Website: http://www.dentistryiq.com/index.html
Facebook, Instagram, and Twitter: @DentistryIQ
This organization's website has separate sections for dentists, assistants, hygienists, and others in the allied dentistry field and has up-to-date news and many informative articles.

National Association of Dental Laboratories (NADL)
325 John Knox Road #L103
Tallahassee, FL 32303
(800) 950-1150
Website: https://nadl.org/home-page.cfm
Facebook: @NADL1951
NADL is the trade association for individuals in the dental laboratory technology industry, including dental laboratory technicians. NADL works to advance the role of the dental lab technician, promote formal education, and administer professional standards for certification.

National Board for Certification in Dental Laboratory Technology (NBC)
325 John Knox Road #L103
Tallahassee, FL 32303
(800) 684-5310
Website: http://www.nbccert.org
An independent board created by the National Association of Dental Laboratories, NBC is responsible for making certain that dental laboratories and technicians adhere to the highest standards and follow all regulations in the industry. NBC approves examinations for the certification program for dental technicians.

Oral Health America
180 North Michigan Avenue, Suite 1150
Chicago, IL 60601
(312) 836-9900
Website: https://oralhealthamerica.org
Facebook: @OralHealthAmerica
Instagram and Twitter: @Smile4Health
This national nonprofit organization promotes oral health across the country by sponsoring school-based educational programs and health education for older adults. They partner with other organizations and advocate for oral health legislation.

FOR FURTHER READING

Brezina, Corona. *Getting a Job in Health Care* (Job Basics: Getting the Job You Need). New York, NY: Rosen Publishing, 2014.

Byers, Ann. *A Career as a Dental Hygienist* (Essential Careers). New York, NY: Rosen Publishing, 2013.

Byers, Ann. *Careers in Dentistry* (Essential Careers). New York, NY: Rosen Publishing, 2018.

Graham, Amy. *Be Smart About Your Career. College, Income, and Careers* (Be Smart About Money and Financial Literacy). New York, NY: Enslow Publishing, 2014.

Henneberg, Susan. *The Vo-Tech Track to Success in Health Care* (Learning a Trade, Preparing for a Career). New York, NY: Rosen Publishing, 2015.

Henry, Kevin. *Battling the Demons of Dental Assisting: How Dental Assistants Can Have an Amazing, Fulfilling Career*. Oceanside, CA: Indie Books International, 2017.

Hubbard, Rita L. *What Degree Do I Need to Pursue a Degree in Health Care?* (The Right Degree for Me). New York, NY: Rosen Publishing, 2015.

Hunsaker, Jennifer. *Dental Hygienists* (Careers in Healthcare). Broomall, PA: Mason Crest, 2018.

Institute for Career Research. *Careers in Dental Laboratory Technology*. N.P.: CreateSpace Independent Publishing Platform, 2015.

Leavitt, Amie Jane. *Jump-Starting a Career in Medical Technology* (Health Care Careers in 2 Years). New York, NY: Rosen Publishing, 2014.

McDowall, Natasha. *Dental Assisting: No Experience Needed—Start on Your Journey to Earning over*

$50,000 a Year. N.P.: CreateSpace Independent Publishing Platform, 2015.

Ratigan, Gerald. *Aced: Superior Interview Skills to Gain an Unfair Advantage to Land Your Dream Job!* N.P: Amazon Digital Services, LLC, 2017.

Sheen, Barbara. *Careers in Health Care* (Exploring Careers). San Diego, CA: ReferencePoint Press, 2014.

BIBLIOGRAPHY

American Dental Association. "Dental Hygienist." Retrieved March 14, 2018. https://www.ada.org/en/education-careers/careers-in-dentistry/dental-team-careers/dental-hygienist.

American Dental Association. "Dental Laboratory Technology." Retrieved March 12, 2018. https://www.ada.org/en/education-careers/careers-in-dentistry/dental-team-careers/dental-laboratory-technology.

Ameritech. "How to Become a Dental Laboratory Technician." 2017. Retrieved March 13, 2018. https://www.ameritech.edu/blog/become-a-dental-lab-technician/.

Best Colleges.com. "Best Online Certificate in Dental Assistance Programs of 2018." Retrieved March 10, 2018. http://www.bestcolleges.com/features/top-online-dental-assistance-certificate-programs.

Best Jobs. "Dental Hygienist Overview." *US News & World Report*, 2017. Retrieved February 20, 2018. https://money.usnews.com/careers/best-jobs/dental-hygienist.

Cargill, Peter. "How to Achieve Success as a Dental Assistant." Dentistry IQ, April 18, 2017. http://www.dentistryiq.com/articles/2017/04/how-to-achieve-success-as-a-dental-assistant.html.

Center for Scientific Information. "Oral Health Topics. Infection Control." ADA Science Institute, American Dental Association, September 12, 2017. http://www.ada.org/en/member-center/oral-health-topics/infection-control-resources.

Decker, Fred. "How to Become a Dental Lab Technician." Career Trend, July 5, 2017. https://careertrend.com/how-14295-become-dental-lab.html

Dental Assistant Training School. "The Top 10 Characteristics of a Successful Dental Assistant." DATS/ Rio Grande Valley, October 18, 2017. https://www.datrainingschool.com/the-top-10-characteristics-of-a-successful-dental-assistant.

Dental Hygienist Salary Jobs. "Top 10 Tools a Dental Hygienist Can't Go Without." Retrieved February 15, 2018. http://www.dentalhygienistsalaryjobs.com/top-10-tools-a-dental-hygienist-cant-go-without.

Elsenpeter, Robert. "5 Ways to Conduct Infection Control Training for Your Office." DPR's Modern Dental Network, December 12, 2017. http://www.dentalproductsreport.com/article/5-ways-conduct-infection-control-training-your-office?page=0,0.

Emmerling, Heidi, and Shirley Gutkowski. "How to Interview for Your First Position as a Dental Hygienist." April 18, 2013. http://www.dentistryiq.com/articles/2013/04/how-to-interview-for-your-first-position-as-a-dental-hygienist.html.

Garlough, Dorothy, RDH, MPA. "Experimenting with Mentoring." RDH, July 10, 2015. http://www.rdhmag.com/articles/print/volume-35/issue-7/columns/experimenting-with-mentoring.html.

Hunter, Tija. "Landing That All-important First Job!" Dentistry IQ, August 22, 2011. http://www.dentistryiq.com/articles/2011/08/landing-that-all-important-first-job-.html.

Kothari, Priya D, DMD. "The Ideal Dental Assistant." *Dental Economics* (DE), November 1, 2004. http://www.dentaleconomics.com/articles/print/volume-94/issue-11/features/the-ideal-dental-assistant.html.

Occupational Outlook Handbook. "Dental Assistants." October 24, 2017. https://www.bls.gov/ooh/healthcare/dental-assistants.htm.

Occupational Outlook Handbook. "Dental Hygienists." October 24, 2017. https://www.bls.gov/ooh/healthcare/dental-hygienists.htm.

Occupational Outlook Handbook. "Dental and Ophthalmic Laboratory Technicians and Medical Appliance Technicians." October 24, 2017. https://www.bls.gov/ooh/production/dental-and-ophthalmic-laboratory-technicians-and-medical-appliance-technicians.htm.

Owen, Jaime. "A Day in the Life of a Dental Assistant." Aol.com, April 20, 2010. https://www.aol.com/2010/04/20/dental-assistant-jobs/.

PayScale, "Dental Hygienist Salary." 2017. https://www.payscale.com/research/US/Job=Dental_Hygienist/Hourly_Rate.

Perry, Doug, and Tracie Perry. "4 Job-hunting Documents Every Dental Hygienist Should Have." Dentistry IQ. July 8, 2015. http://www.dentistryiq.com/articles/2015/07/four-job-hunting-documents-every-dental-hygienist-should-have-tracie-doug-parry.html.

Siebert, Karen. "A Day in the Life of a Dental Hygienist." Retrieved December 2, 2017. http://dept.clcillinois.edu/biodv/healthlibrary/pdf/life_DentalHygienist.pdf.

Smith, Jacquelyn. "Externships: What They Are and Why They're Important." *Forbes*, May 30, 2013. https://www.forbes.com/sites/jacquelynsmith/2013/05/30/externships-what-they-are-and-why-theyre-important/#d5765d05100c.

Vavrosky, Kara. "First Day on the Job? 5 Things to Do during Your First 100 Days in a New Dental Office." RDH, June 12, 2015. http://www.rdhmag.com/articles/print/volume-35/issue-6/columns/first-day-on-the-job.html.

Vista College. "What's in a Smile? A Day in the Life of a Dental Assistant." April 22, 2015. http://www.vistacollege.edu/blog/careers/whats-in-a-smile-a-day-in-the-life-of-a-dental-assistant.

Watson, Eva M. "The Job Interview." RDH, July 1, 2010. http://www.rdhmag.com/articles/print/volume-30/issue-7/features/the-job-interview.html.

INDEX

About the Author

Carol Hand has a PhD in zoology. She has taught college biology and written biology assessments for national assessment companies. Hand has also written middle and high school science curricula for a national company and science books for young adults, including several on medical and health topics such as genetics, food allergies, anxiety disorders, and vaccines.

Photo Credits

Cover (figure) OLJ Studio/Shutterstock.com; cover (background) Luckyraccoon/Shutterstock.com; back cover, p. 1 (background graphic) HunThomas/Shutterstock.com; pp. 4–5 (background) and interior pages 279photo Studio/Shutterstock.com; p. 5 © iStockphoto .com/AntonioGuillem; p. 8 Sirtravelalot/Shutterstock.com; pp. 9, 13 Romaset/Shutterstock.com; pp. 11, 52 Lucidio Studio, Inc./Moment/ Getty Images; p. 17 Johner Images/Getty Images; p. 19 Malorny/ Moment/Getty Images; p. 22 Lucian Coman/Shutterstock.com; p. 25 Tim Brown/The Image Bank/Getty Images; p. 27 Roberto Machado Noa/LightRocket/Getty Images; p. 28 Tom Kelley/Archive Photos/ Getty Images; p. 31 Bloomberg/Getty Images; p. 34 Echo/Juice Images/Getty Images; p. 36 Monty Rakusen/Cultura/Getty Images; p. 40 Moxie Productions/Blend Images/Getty Images; p. 42 ESB Professional/Shutterstock.com; p. 45 Douglas Graham/CQ-Roll Call Group/Getty Images; p. 47 Alpa Prod/Shutterstock.com; pp. 55, 60 Wavebreakmedia/Shutterstock.com; p. 56 Andy Dean Photography/ Shutterstock.com; p. 59 BSIP/Universal Images Group/Getty Images.

Design: Michael Moy; Layout: Ellina Litmanovich; Senior Editor: Kathy Kuhtz Campbell; Photo Researcher: Sherri Jackson